ASTHMA A

Dr Paul Sherwood, consu........ ...., trained at Cambridge Univers.., and the Westminster Hospital. After achieving a degree in medicine he worked as a house surgeon at Westminster Hospital, and later at Barts before becoming a consultant at a number of hospitals.

Dr Sherwood set up his own private clinic in London where he has been developing his own form of physical medicine over a period of 40 years.

BY THE SAME AUTHOR
The Back and Beyond
The Heart Revolution

ASTHMA AND BEYOND

Dr Paul Sherwood

ARROW

Published by Arrow Books in 1995

1 3 5 7 9 10 8 6 4 2

First published in the United Kingdom by
Arrow Books Limited
20 Vauxhall Bridge Road, London, SW1V 2SA

Random House Australia (Pty) Limited
20 Alfred Street, Milsons Point, Sydney,
New South Wales 2061, Australia

Random House New Zealand Limited
18 Poland Road, Glenfield
Auckland 10, New Zealand

Random House South Africa (Pty) Limited
PO Box 337, Bergvlei, South Africa

Random House UK Limited Reg. No. 954009

A CIP catalogue record for this book is available from the British
Library

ISBN 0 09 955231 0

Phototypeset by Intype, London
Printed and Bound in Great Britain by
Cox & Wyman Ltd, Reading, Berkshire

To all the people whom I love for, without them, what would be the purpose of living?

ACKNOWLEDGEMENTS

Once again, I have to thank Mary Atkinson for her tireless energy and patience when translating my thoughts into an orderly and readable form. Even more am I grateful for her endless enthusiasm which has kept my flagging spirits going on so many occasions. Her husband, Richard and long suffering children Emma and Lizzie also deserve medals – I am working on it. My family put up with me with an air of amused tolerance, but are always willing to read something to see if it makes sense or to stop what they are doing to help me find the 'perfect' word to suite the occasion. They all deserve a slap up dinner. A special mention to my secretary Wendy, who has endlessly rearranged my practice at a second's notice to liberate me for some chore or other to do with the book. My thanks to my other secretary Annabel, the lightening typist who has typed long passages out from my illegible script before the paper has settled on her desk. Also to all my staff who have worked extra hard to allow me to prosecute this awesome task. And last but not least – to my friend Peter who thought of the perfect title 'A Breath of Fresh Air' for the book – but which was unfortunately rejected by the publishers. And lastly my thanks to Francesca Zeissl who has read the manuscript and ironed out the wrinkles.

CONTENTS

AUTHORS NOTE

Some years ago a professor of medicine came to see me for treatment to his back. On his third visit he remarked in a rather peeved tone of voice that he had been talking to a patient in the waiting room who had asthma. The professor wanted to know what possible connection there could be between his back trouble and the other patient's asthma. How could I treat both conditions when they appeared to be so far removed from each other? Similarly, having already written one book, *The Back and Beyond*, which deals with the back itself and a number of diseases associated with the back, and then *The Heart Revolution*, which is concerned with coronary thrombosis, it might seem strange that I should suddenly write a third book on a further set of apparently dissimilar diseases. The answer is that my approach to the treatment of a particular complaint is quite different to the attitude generally adopted in the world of conventional medicine. The tendency is for a person to become a specialist in a certain part of the body such as the eye or the foot, the abdomen or chest. The expert knows every sort of illness that affects his chosen part of the body whether it be malformations, infections, injury or tumours. The chest specialist, for example, deals with a wide variety of diseases in the one particular spot in the body.

To my mind, it makes far more sense to deal with one

particular type of disease, and then whatever part and function of the body it affects. This seems a much more logical approach as diseases have a bad habit of not sticking accurately to anatomical boundaries. A doctor who specializes in one part of the body may not realize that a different disease somewhere else could be causing the problem in that area. An arthritic joint, for example, can be caused by an infected tonsil. I, on the other hand, specialize in the two main defence mechanisms of the body and anything that may go wrong with them in any part of the body: these are the lymphatic system and the sympathetic nerve system.

The latter is the subject of my two previous books, the former is dealt with here. Although the two systems are very efficient, they can malfunction, for various reasons, many of which are to do with the fact that our civilized way of life is very different to the living conditions for which the body was designed. My treatment aims to restore the normal function of the defective defence and repair mechanism and so help the body do its own job. This is the common link in my practice and explains why I treat back problems, sinus problems, arthritis, migraine right through to indigestion, as all these have the common factor of being caused by faults in these systems.

The professor understood the force of my arguments. However he said that because they cut across the current approach and attitude of the profession, my ideas may be sadly misunderstood. I hope that the publication of three books has helped to add cohesion and clarity to my theories.

FOREWORD

'A Breath of Fresh Air' seemed the perfect title for this book as it reflected the clearing of the air that I have tried to achieve on the subject of the lymph system as this is generally poorly understood. It did not, however, sufficiently suggest the content of the book, so *Asthma and Beyond* was thought to be a more suitable title. Many other diseases, however, are also caused by faulty functioning of the lymph system.

The lymph system is one of the main defence and repair mechanisms in the body. It is often thought to be trouble-free except when it is involved with diseases like leukaemia. However, this is curious when one considers that the tonsils and appendix, which are a major part of the lymph system, are notorious for causing both chronic and acute problems. So surely the rest of the lymph system may not be so totally blameless either?

Asthma and Beyond explains how distressing diseases such as asthma, eczema, sinus trouble and cystitis are caused by malfunctions of the lymph system. So too are many other debilitating ailments including bronchitis, laryngitis, arthritis, middle and inner ear troubles. As soon as the lymph system is restored to working order then the disease can usually be greatly or even completely relieved.

Over the past 40 years I have treated many people with conditions associated with a damaged lymph system.

13

Many of these patients had either been told that little or nothing could be done to help, or that they would need to take drugs probably for the rest of their lives. By using physical medicine to treat the ailing lymph system, I can nearly always help a patient enjoy a fit and healthy life free from pain, discomfort and a reliance on drugs.

Patients come from all over the world and there seems to be a universal lack of understanding of the lymph system. When I explain the function of the system and how a blockage in its mechanism has caused their ailment, it is rewarding to feel the sense of relief that accompanies a new insight into the workings of the body. Equipped with this knowledge, they are then able to play a major part in their own or their child's recovery.

Management At Home

Problems with the lymph system usually start at a very young age even though in some cases the main symptoms do not occur until much later in life. So this book is particularly aimed at parents and teachers as many of the causes can so easily be avoided. It also shows parents how to give home-based, simple, safe treatment to the lymph system if the child has already started to suffer.

Some symptoms may be obvious, such as constant infections, sore throats and bronchial troubles but others are not usually associated with illness. A bad-tempered, inattentive and rude child, for example, may be punished for bad behaviour when what he really needs is treatment to his defective lymph nodes. In such instances I have always found that, once the fault in the lymph system has been corrected, the change in personality is quite overwhelming.

Many diseases such as asthma are considered hereditary and parents all too often resign themselves to the fact that their child will suffer – but this need not be. Certainly, a child may have a tendency to the disease, but that can almost always be overcome by taking appropriate action early in the child's life. The book contains detailed preventative measures so that parents can take an active role in the management of their children's health. The recommendations, which you can practise at home, are very simple and dramatic in effect.

But to participate fully in your child's recovery, you must first of all understand the cause of the problem. The book illustrated with diagrams, therefore, gives a detailed explanation of the lymph system.

The Drainage System of the Body

The lymph system is the sewerage system of the entire body, forming an extremely efficient mechanism for dealing with infection, damage or foreign bodies in the tissue spaces. Its function is integrally linked with the circulation of blood. Briefly, blood is carried away from the heart through the arteries to the capillaries where fluid diffuses from the blood into the tissue spaces taking with it essential supplies and oxygen. This fluid then diffuses back into the other end of the capillaries, carrying with it carbon dioxide and waste products, and then flows into the veins.

Lymph vessels, or lymphatics as they are called, play an important part in this process if the tissues become infected, or if there is tissue damage or a foreign body present. The lymphatics are ducts which, unlike the arteries and veins, open directly into the tissue spaces. Thus they are able to carry away not only tissue fluids, which increase under these circumstances, but also minute foreign bodies such as bacteria.

The tissue fluid, known as lymph once it passes into the

lymphatics, flows through a network of lymph nodes on its way back to the veins and these filter out and destroy any dead cells, bacteria, viruses and other foreign bodies. Each set of lymph nodes is concerned with draining a particular area of the body.

Defense Against Bacteria

It is in the lymph nodes that we produce antibodies against foreign proteins, such as those found in invading bacteria or viruses, carried to them from the tissue spaces. The tonsils, adenoids and appendix are all part of the lymph system. They form the first line of defence against infection. What is more, they are able to culture bacteria in their own 'test-tubes' and produce antibodies against them in order to protect us in advance against all these bacteria and viruses should they invade in the future.

Obstructing the Drainage

Under ideal conditions, the lymph system is an extremely efficient network for dealing with infection rapidly, completely, and often permanently. Chapter 1 shows how the lymph nodes can be overloaded with infection and debris and become partially blocked. This obstructs the flow of lymph through the nodes and causes back-pressure of fluid, in the part of the lymph system which drains into them causing a number of problems such as: swollen membranes causing lowered resistance to infection and obstruction of the passages they line such as from the sinuses and the middle ear: and the inability to throw off an infection.

However, in Chapter 2 we look at how 'advances' in modern living, such as wearing clothes, heating our houses and processing food, have gone a long way to weakening our lymph systems. Our huge population means that we come into contact with far more infection than our bodies are originally designed to cope with, particularly in the first years of life. Under these circumstances, the efficient workings of the lymph system can easily be thwarted.

Treating the Problem

Much of the treatment can be home-based but when this is not sufficient to treat the problem, it is necessary to obtain professional help. In my treatment there is little place for the drugs which are commonly used. The mainstay of the treatment is physical medicine using ultrasonic waves (long-wave sound is even better), massage and surged faradism. These break up the debris that has collected in the lymph nodes and pump a flow of fluid through them much as you would use a rubber plunger to clear tea-leaves that have blocked the drain in your sink. As the blockage is removed and the drainage improves, the lymph system becomes able to do its job. The patient not only feels better but also gains an increased resistance to infections.

The equipment and knowledge needed for the widespread use of the treatment is available, but at present the resources are not used in this manner. All the necessary information, instructions and diagrams for local practitioners to give the treatment can be found in Chapter 7. However, it is important to realize that there can come a time when the system irretrievably breaks down and treatment alone is not enough.

This applies particularly to the tonsils and appendix which are in the front line of attack and can be destroyed by the bacteria they are trying to eliminate. Chapter 3 clarifies the confusion between enlarged tonsils, which may be working hard to ward off infection, and damaged tonsils, which must be removed, and gives firm guidelines for the ultimate decision regarding removal of the damaged organ. The appendix is also considered in detail as, again, there is sometimes doubt as to what should be its fate. Decisions are particularly important because, if it is not removed when it should be, then it can cause prolonged ill-health of a kind not normally associated with a damaged appendix.

It is my hope that this book will bring an altogether better understanding of the lymph system and its associated illnesses.

1

WASTE DISPOSAL WHAT CAN GO WRONG?

Obstruction of the Drains

One of the main roles of the lymph system is to act as the sewerage system within the body. So, in order to look at what can go wrong, a useful analogy, although a rather unsavoury one, is to compare the lymph drainage with the soil pipe for a block of flats, with the toilets in each flat representing the various tissues drained by a lymph node. The lymph node can be compared to an inspection manhole where blockages can occur. Under normal circumstances this system services all the flats efficiently and is able to cope with fairly heavy demands.

But, there are certain circumstances when conditions may slow down the drainage and even bring it to a complete halt. Perhaps the most unlikely happening, but still a possibility, would be that the actual pipe itself is damaged. In the same way, operations or an injury, particularly one to the neck, may involve cutting through the lymph ducts and this might upset the free drainage through these channels. Although the body can grow new lymph vessels, the effects of the initial blockage still need to be sorted out before they cause longer term problems.

It is far more common, however, for the system to be effected either by a constant input of debris from the toilets, which slowly and by degrees starts to block the

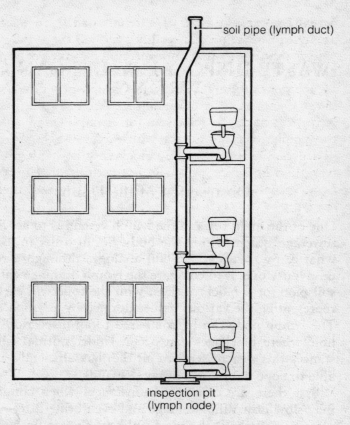

soil pipe (lymph duct)

inspection pit
(lymph node)

Figure 1

inspection pit; or by a sudden barrage of items from one toilet that obstructs it more-or-less straightaway. In the case of the lymph system, the partial blockage is brought about by either a series of low-grade infections, which are commonly found in the bladder or the throat, or a continuous very low-grade infection such as athlete's foot; or by a very intense infection, usually in the throat or lung. As these latter both cover a very large area (the lung

20

actually covers the size of a tennis court) an excessive amount of infection can readily overload the system.

In the same way that an inspection pit may get partially blocked, a group of lymph nodes can become obstructed by the debris brought in by the lymph generated in the infected area. A series of minor sore throats or one particularly virulent throat infection, for example, may overload the lymph nodes in the neck which drain the throat. These nodes then become partially blocked. It is worth stressing here that the lymph nodes do not get obstructed on their own, it is always due to the debris brought into them by the lymph.

Just as a blocked inspection pit will cause the offending toilet to overflow because water cannot drain away, so a partially obstructed lymph node will prevent the tissue fluid from flowing away causing the tissues to fill with fluid and upset the tissue circulation in the catchment area. Such a situation has repercussions throughout the whole system. Imagine, if someone flushed the toilet on the ground floor of a block of flats with unsuitable items, blocking the inspection pit; then when someone in the top floor flat flushes their toilet, there will be back pressure which will force the waste to come out in the WC pans not only in the ground floor but also in other flats.

A similar process occurs in the body when a lymph node has become partially blocked. If, for example, a person has had a series of bad sore throats, then other areas sharing the same lymph drainage such as the ears, sinuses or eyes can be effected causing their membranes to become swollen. This can have varying consequences.

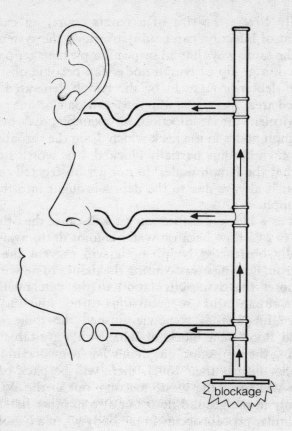

Figure 2

Swollen Membranes

Membranes are usually very thin indeed, being one cell thick, square and flat – they are in fact called 'pavement membranes'. However, under adverse circumstances the cells can multiply and swell to become enormously thick – even reaching around a quarter of an inch (60 mm). This is because the diminished tissue circulation does not

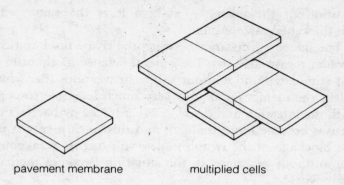

pavement membrane   multiplied cells

Figure 3

provide the cells with enough nourishment so in their weakened state they will multiply to form a thick wall between the bacteria invading from the outside and the tissues. Just as an apple tree produces huge numbers of apples as a survival mechanism if the roots or bark become seriously damaged.

This enlarged wall is intended to provide protection, but it means in actual fact that the outside layer of the membrane is much further away from the protection of defenders and nutrients in the tissue circulation. As the army of white cells is prevented from reaching the bacteria it does not have the chance to attack and carry them away in the lymph vessels. Instead, the bacteria start to grow in the outer part of the thick wall using it for protection.

The situaion is rather like a village that has a defensive wall around it. The villagers decide they need extra protection so they thicken the wall in an attempt to keep the invaders out. However a thicker wall, possibly up to half a mile across, means that the invading army can gather on the top without the villagers even being aware. Now the invaders can attack with every chance of success. And so the wall actually weakens rather than strengthens the position of the village – and so it is the same with the thickened membrane.

The increased distance between the tissue fluid and the invader means also that the general defence mechanism is not stimulated and without sufficient weapons (i.e. white cells), the membrane is also very much less able to cope with the infection and throw it off. Attacks by bacteria or viruses become more frequent and this in turn speeds up the blockage of the lymph nodes, still further weakening the antibody response so the situation becomes increasingly worse.

In the Author's Note, it was noted that several seemingly unconnected areas are often drained by the same lymph nodes. So, as the diagram shows, the back pressure of the fluid caused by partially blocked lymph nodes can spread up tubes leading to other parts of the body and effect the drainage from other membranes. An irritation in the nose could, for example, affect the drainage from the sinuses or middle ear. Should that happen these membranes will also thicken making them vulnerable to attack by any bacteria or viruses that settle in the area. The congestion will also bring with it other specific problems (which will be discussed in Chapters 3 to 7); but in general terms:

- The reduced antibody response means that the person is likely to succumb to any kind of infection more readily and take longer to shrug it off.
- The repair mechanism will be affected so any, cuts, wounds or operations will not heal so quickly.
- The excess fluid which cannot drain away may cause swelling, particularly in the ankles.

Unblocking the System

The conventional approach to treating an infection is to bring in extra weapons, such as an antibiotic, to help the failing army win this particular battle. The disadvantage of this is that it encourages the army to become careless about maintaining all its equipemnt as it realizes it will have outside rescue in the event of any other crisis. It may also make less powerful enemies more prone to attack as they see the run-down state of the defence.

My approach is to enable the body to look after its own defence unaided by reorganizing and retraining the army; thus not only is it able to cope with the particular emergency but it will be much more efficient on any future occasion and its very strength will act as a major deterrent to aggressors. My treatment therefore aims to improve the drainage of the tissue fluids through the lymph sewers thus reducing the back pressure or traffic jam in the tissue spaces. This restores a proper tissue circulation and reduces the size of the swollen membrane which has immediate benefits for the present complaint and also improves the future health of the patient by increasing both resistance to infection and the ability to throw it off. Once drainage to the lymph nodes is restored:

- The health of the tissues themselves improves.
- Dead cells, bacteria and debris can be removed.
- The supply of white cells and antibodies to the area is restored.
- The infecting organism is now taken to the lymph nodes resulting in an increase in the production of white cells and antibodies which are transported to the affected area.

Helping the Body Heal Itself

The treatment involves physical medicine using a combination of tools depending on the individual complaint and the accessibility of the area concerned. In most cases the part of the body involved can be treated as well as the remote part of the associated drainage system. However, in certain instances such as the middle ear, only the drainage system can be accessed. The treatment employs conventional physiotherapy but modified to a totally different use. It should therefore be possible to obtain it locally from any qualified therapist. The treatment is fortunately not only painless but actually pleasant. Specific details for each disease will be dicussed alongside the particular complaint in later chapters, but the general principle of the treatment involves:

- **Massage** to the lymph nodes which helps break up the debris and improves the flow of tissue fluid through the nodes. The massage should be moderately firm with the fingers in a rotating movement, but always in the general direction of the drainage, i.e. towards the heart. It should be firm enough to be really felt but not to be painful. If the lymph nodes are particularly tender then this massage can be uncomfortable but it should never hurt. It only needs a few minutes and is a manoeuvre that can easily be carried out at home – either on your child or yourself – once or twice daily until the lymph nodes return to their normal size.

- **Ultrasonic Waves** are used to vibrate the affected lymph nodes. This helps break up the debris making it easier for it to be removed piecemeal or to be converted to soluble products. Ultrasonic waves are sound waves that hit a far higher note than a human or even a dog can hear. They are thought to speed up the affect of any chemical reaction, so that the lymph nodes are able to carry out their functions much more efficiently. The new long wave sound therapy seems even more beneficial in most cases. Fortunately, massage alone is so effective that the end result is probably as good but the ultrasonic achieves it more rapidly.

- **Surged Faradism** has the effect of making the muscles contract and relax rhythmically and simultaneously as a whole group. This is achieved by applying surged faradic stimulation to the skin over the nerve which supplies the muscles, or sometimes over the muscles themselves, to obtain a graded rhythm of contractions. As the muscles contract they will drive the fluid out of themselves and nearby tissues into the lymph ducts; as they relax, they will all refill with tissue fluid that is replaced from the arterial system, ready to be pumped down through the lymph vessels once again. This form of treatment works by clearing the lymph nodes and improving the drainage through them much the same as you would clear the drain of your kitchen sink if it becomes blocked with tea leaves. You take a rubber plunger to propel the water down the pipe in explosive bursts which break up the mass of leaves and help to carry it off. In the same way, fluid in the tissue spaces is driven in one co-ordinated pulse down through the lymph vessels that go to the affected nodes. This is brought about by making as many of the muscles as possible in the catchment area contract at the same time.

People vary enormously in all respects, not least in the

number of treatments they require. Obviously, a guideline is needed but the amount depends not only on the severity and extent of the problem plus the make-up of the patient, but also on the skill of the therapist. There is usually a worthwhile improvement early on with the treatment but most patients need somewhere between five and twenty sessions to reduce the clinical signs (symptoms are that which the patient notices, signs are that which the doctor discovers) to an acceptable level. The symptoms may often take several months after this fully to resolve.

- **Drugs** may be very helpful in addition to the physical medicine.

Anti-Inflammatory Drugs

In painful conditions produced by an inflammatory process, and rarely in infections, anti-inflammatory drugs help by greatly reducing the substance called prostaglandin. This substance is secreted locally in the tissues and designed to improve their ability to cope with any emergency but which so hopelessly overdoes the reaction that not only does it finally impede recovery but the effect of it almost become an illness in itself. Imagine a town in a major country which has a small riot. Hysterical telephone messages to the capital result in a major invasion of the town by the army. Streets are blocked by tanks and the troops, road blocks interfere with distribution, special police arrest all numbers of innocent citizens, builders, supply and refuse vehicles are brought to a standstill, in the chaos the rioters cannot be found, the whole town begins to decay, people starve and disease spreads. The effect is infinitely worse than the original riot. If the telephone calls for help can be reduced to a moderate level, then only a few troops and police will be kept in the town, and they will be able to deal with the riot much more easily and without disrupting the rest of the town. Neutralizing most of the prostaglandin and cutting back the messages is effectively what anti-inflammatory drugs do.

Antibiotics

A major advance in modern medicine is the use of antibiotics. In my view they are some of the most valuable drugs in the pharmacopoeia, but because of their enormous power and effectiveness they are also one of the most abused. They are only useful if they are going to relieve a distressing or damaging infection or one that is a threat to life or future health. As a routine treatment for people with minor infections they give extremely unsatisfactory results and only act to weaken the body's own powers of defence and repair. If children are given antibiotics for every infection they catch then their body's own defences never really get a chance to get going and they do not form the wide range of antibodies needed to defend them against future infections.

I saw Arabella when she was 12. She had constant sore throats, and some accompanied by a very high temperature. On each occasion she had been given antibiotic treatment which did relieve the problem within a few days but unfortunately in some weeks she went down with yet another attack. She had got rather large, nasty looking tonsils and I arranged to have these taken out. Arabella felt better for a while but when she had another sore throat she went back to her doctor, who prescribed more antibiotic treatment.

I had noticed that three other youngsters who were my patients had all been looked after by the same doctor who had prescribed antibiotics for every throat infection. Against this there was another rather elderly doctor who had a strong objection to antibiotics and who had only

29

referred one patient to me. This child, Peter, aged eight, came to me because he was having problems with his ears and the doctor wondered if the enlarged lymph nodes might mean trouble later in his life.

In the past Peter had suffered a sore throat but it had gone away without the use of antibiotics in about five days. He had been fit for six years before he went down with another infection. Peter obviously had a strong lymph system and as the enlarged lymph nodes were soft I was sure that they were merely working hard to try and keep the child fit. We did nothing and the lymph nodes all went down without any treatment. Peter has remained fit and well.

A research study published in the medical journals contrasted a thousand children who were treated with antibiotics when they caught a sore throat and a thousand that were not. These children were all around the same age with somewhat similar types of sore throat. On average those who were not treated with antibiotics had sore throats for four days – the recurrence rate was 3%. The children who were treated with antibiotics had an average recovery rate of three days but the recurrence rate was 68%. It seems therefore that antibiotics are not a first choice for the treatment of sore throats. Possibly it is best to reserve them for: when the infection is serious and accompanied by a high temperature; if the ear is involved; or some other complication occurs that needs to be eliminated quickly.

One of the problems with the use of antibiotics is that there is a sad misunderstanding as to what is a course of the drug. A patient who is given enough tablets for five or seven days is often satisfied that this is the correct amount to cure his immediate problem – even though he is not free of the trouble at the end of the period. Antibiotics work by being a kind of anaesthetic on the bacteria, slowing them down so giving the body an opportunity to mop up the helpless victims.

The bacteria within a single colony have widely variable powers of resistance. This means that in the early days of taking antibiotics the patient loses the very weakest, followed by the weak and then finally the strongest strains of the organism. It follows from this that if an antibiotic is abandoned before it has done its job completely, the patient will be left with only the most virulent strains.

When the antibiotic is stopped at this point, the bacteria that remain will begin to multiply, replacing those that were killed, so the whole of the new infection will consist of the most virulent strain – which is also, of course, much more resistant to the antibiotic. A course of antibiotics is, therefore, whatever is needed to eliminate the infection and should not be numbered in days. It might require five days, three weeks or, in rare cases, even a year or more. It should also be given in the strongest safe dosage to eliminate the most resistant bacteria as rapidly and completely as possible.

I saw Pippa when she was 17. At the age of five she had flu and from then on had had a large number of sore throats. When she was 11 she had her tonsils out but she still had catarrh with sinus trouble and a low grade bronchitis. When she caught a cold it went straight to her chest and she remained very chesty for some weeks. She had been having ear trouble for two years before I saw her for ear ache accompanied by more infection in the sinuses.

A test showed that Pippa had become rather deaf in her left ear. On examination she had a number of enlarged lymph nodes in both sides of the neck particularly just below the ear. The drums of both ears were affected and her throat was somewhat red. This inflammation continued as far down her throat as could reasonably be seen. She

31

had treatment to the lymph nodes and although this did improve her condition, she was still having earache and bronchial infections with a sort of asthmatic wheeze when it was at its worst.

Finally, I decided to put her onto an antibiotic to clear this infection and I kept her on it for nearly six months. During this time the infection cleared and it stayed at a satisfactory level. However, as soon as she stopped taking the antibiotic, she became catarrhal again and started wheezing. Eventually, Pippa was able to give up the antibiotics and when I saw her a year later she told me that she had suffered no recurrence of the problem.

Pippa's experience highlights the fact that there is no set dose of antibiotics – each patient needs the right amount to clear the infection completely. A doctor will usually give you a quantity that is a reasonable estimate of what may be needed and will then want to see you before this amount has run out. He can then decide whether you need to continue the course and, on the basis of the previous performance, how long it may now take. He will, of course, wish to review the situation at the end of the further extension in case the dosage should still prove to have been inadequate. So long as there are no adverse effects, such as allergies to the antibiotic or other necessary bacteria in the body being killed by the antibiotics, then keeping a patient on antibiotics for a long period of time is a completely safe practice.

Unfortunately, unlike the antibodies produced by the body, antibiotics have no magic property of eliminating only undesirable bacteria. They will also work on other vulnerable groups and this can include some of the essential bacteria in the body, especially in the bowel. Many people, when taking antibiotics, become deficient in Vitamin B and some of the natural bacterial flora, which may lead to depression or even a serious enteritis, caused by a multiplication of one of the other bacterium or fungi already present. Normally the bacterium of the gut tend to compete with the fungal inhabitants for food. If the bacteria are removed then there is considerably more food available for the fungus; for example, Candida. This is then able to multiply unopposed and cause irritation. It is widely thought that taking Vitamin B with some antibiotics helps to prevent this. The reintroduction of bacteria by swallowing missing cultures may also be helpful in restoring health after a course of antibiotics.

- **Dietary Advice** may also be appropriate. Food sensitivities come about from the natural reaction of an inflamed stomach to foods that it finds particularly hard to deal with. To prevent further aggravation the body secretes a huge quantity of cortisole. One of the functions of this substance is to protect the body from irritants; it reduces inflammation (that is why it is used for treating arthritis) and also cuts down the capillary circulation in the area. Unfortunately, the cortisole is soon used up reaching a level well below normal. This results in an increase of the capillary circulation all over the body so that any catarrhal condition is greatly exaggerated.

The most common culprits causing food sensitivities are cow's milk, gluten (which is one of the substances in white flour), gelatine and coffee. There are approved ways to test for sensitivities such as skin tests but the snag with almost all of these is that they only relate to the actual tissue tested. Skin tests, therefore, are of little value in telling you what your intestines react to. Blood tests are very accurate but extremely expensive. Also if so much as one food substance causing a sensitivity is left out, which is easily done, the whole test becomes useless. There is also a variety of less scientific methods employed for assessing food sensitivities. I have had patients assessed by many of these over a period of time and I am a little doubtful as to their total efficacy. The results always seem to come back much the same with every patient i.e. that they are sensitive to white flour, milk products, yeast, sugar and coffee. Avoiding these substances helps about 75% of the sufferers. If the patient is not one of the lucky 75% he does not seem able to be helped by the practitioner any more and is advised to experiment himself to find any other allergies that may be present.

I now advise people to use their instinct. You can usually tell if you or your child is particularly sensitive to a food because either you don't like it or, much more commonly, you are excessively keen on the offending food or drink. This is because, when the sensitivity is well developed, as soon as you take the food on board, the body counteracts its effect with a tremendous secretion of cortisole. This gives you an immense feeling of well-being so you associate that food with feeling exceptionally good. As the effect of the cortisole dies off the feeling changes to one of lowness and depression. Your subconscious immediately wants another biscuit or slice of white bread, or whatever the offending substance, to give you a lift.

Breast feeding your child, if it is possible, can waive a lot of problems in his early years. All too often, cows milk is given as a substitute for breast milk but the body doesn't always tolerate it well. Milk is so widely considered as an essential ingredient of a wholesome diet that many mothers become anxious if their children don't like it. However, children have an incredible ability to choose the foods that best suit their bodies. This point is illustrated by an experiment carried out in America some years ago. It involved 9000 orphan children in institutions, aged between 1 and 7, who were divided into three groups, for about ten years. The first group was fed on a diet specially devised by top dieticians and paediatricians; the second group was fed on an average diet; and the third group could eat exactly what they liked from a selection of everyday foods. They were given twelve choices in little dishes in front of them but could ask for anything that was not present. They could eat as much as they liked of whatever they liked. There was no control over their intake except that sugar was missing from the diet. There were two reasons for this, first that sugar is very difficult to come by in any quantity in nature – we get it either from sugar cane or beet – both of these are grown specifically for the sugar industry. Without these crops it would be very difficult to have any appreciable quantity in our diet. Secondly in very small quantities sugar is an almost perfect food. These two facts mean that our discriminatory sense does not work very well and we have little built in limitation of its intake. As is well known, large quantities of sugar upset the sugar/fat metabolism and cause a number of problems, including hardening of the arteries.

The end result of the experiment showed that there was little difference between the first and second groups but that the third group was by far the most healthy. Indeed, even the radiologist could tell the difference between it and the other two groups by studying the growth and density of the bones.

When the researchers tried to analyse the diet of the third group of children there was one overwhelming conclusion – no analysis was possible. All the children ate different things and they all had fads that frequently changed. Some would eat only one thing, some a few and some many different foods. The actual diet of each child was totally dependent on the particular day and displayed no pattern at all. The only clear result was that milk proved extremely unpopular, with few touching it at all, so clearly it is not necessary for a healthy diet.

Left to their own devices then, children will eat what they need when they need it. The only big exception is sugar which is an acquired taste developed as a habit at a young age when adults start indulging children with sweets. Once you develop a 'sweet tooth' it's very hard to break the habit. Unfortunately, sugar is also the ideal fuel for bacteria and yeasts (fungi). If you have a large quantity of sugar in your mouth then it becomes a breeding ground for bacteria. Eating sweet foods encourages all the bacteria present in your body to multiply, as dental advertisements make only too clear.

Diet Supplements

Patients almost always need extra vitamins and trace elements. When I first started to write this book in the 1950s people were saying that our food met all out dietetic requirements and that it was ridiculous to give supplements which could even be harmful. However, more recent research has shown that children and adults actually do much better with additional vitamins.

Even though your diet contains all the vitamins you need, you cannot always assume that you absorb enough of them. Your body may destroy, or use up, particularly large quantities of the vitamins; or you may have an absorption problem. With petrol stations in such rich supply you would think it impossible for anyone to let their tank run dry; yet the AA say their biggest reason for being called out is because people have run out of petrol.

You simply cannot argue that just because there is petrol everywhere that everyone has enough. It is the same with the body.

Even though a diet has an adequate supply of vitamins and minerals, the body may not absorb enough. For example, large quantities of alcohol or hot spices may cause a gastritis, which can affect absorption of Vitamin B, magnesium and other trace substances. People with back trouble and catarrhal conditions may suffer from the same problem. Anxiety states, infection and depression often result in a massive destruction of Vitamin B and the excretion of magnesium; if the person has absorption problems the body is not able to replace them readily.

The vitamins which usually need to be supplemented are Vitamins A, B and C. I believe that children and adults should take recommended daily doses of cod liver oil or halibut oil capsules to ensure adequate Vitamin A and D. It is also important for children to have extra Vitamin B throughout their growing life. It is best for children to take Vitamin B in liquid form. Adults, particularly over the age of forty-five, should choose synthetic formulations of Vitamin B, as natural sources so often contain yeast which can be upsetting.

Even if you eat plenty of fresh fruit you cannot be sure you are getting enough Vitamin C as I believe that this essential vitamin is often missing when fruit is artificially ripened. It's almost impossible to take too much Vitamin C but I would recommend about 1 to 2 gms a day for adults, with an increase to some 3 or 4 gms a day if you have an infection. A child of 6 stone (44 kg) needs about half a gram a day; and a child of 3 stone (22 kg) should take a quarter of a gram. If your child finds it hard to take a vitamin tablet and it cannot be obtained as a fluid, then an effective method is to crush it up into a powder and using a syringe to blow it into his mouth.

Many people are lacking in essential minerals and it is surprising how much better you can feel simply by taking a mineral supplement. However, you do need to be careful. When I asked a patient recently if she took any extra vitamins or minerals she put 27 bottles on my table, each one labelled for a particular purpose: stopping painful periods, enhancing purity of skin, preventing colds and so on. All the bottles contained much the same minerals and as a result she was taking a serious overdose which meant she was spending a great deal of money and solving nothing. Trace elements are nearly all metals or metalloids. These are poisons if taken in excess so your body has an in-built mechanism to prevent you from absorbing too much. However, it cannot distinguish between each particular substance; it works according to the total amount. When a critical level is reached your body stops absorbing any of them at all. So by taking too much of one mineral you may be missing out on all the other essential trace elements. I would recommend taking one supplement which contains all the necessary trace elements. The only exception is zinc which is probably best taken separately, perhaps at night, as it tends to react with the others and then may not be absorbed.

Sympathetic Nerve Upsets

As has been explained in *The Back and Beyond*, back injuries in the thoracic (chest) area often cause a water-logging of the sympathetic nerve computers, or ganglia as they are called. This results in a low sympathetic drive and produces a number of symptoms. Tiredness and indigestion are two of the most common. A low sympathetic drive can be a significant factor in causing food sensitivities and absorption difficulties. It needs to be considered as a possible component when investigating these problems in a patient. If this is the fault, treatment to the back will be needed, otherwise the patient will never become completely well.

Lifestyle Advice is perhaps one of the most valuable parts of the treatment. It took a million years to evolve a being to exist in the conditions of primitive man. Civilization has turned almost every facet of this existence upside down so advice on helping the body to cope with the very artificial circumstances of our present lifestyle is supremely important. Dealing with this vital part of the treatment needs the space of the whole of the next chapter.

2

A NEW LOOK AT OUR MODERN LIFE STYLE

We have so taken for granted the benefits of modern civilization with our houses and clothes to protect us from the elements and the food industry to provide us with safe eating and drinking, that this chapter may come as quite a shock to many readers when they find that these 'advances' are actually the cause of many health problems. Although these problems may not become evident until later in life, they actually start at a very young age when a child has little control over his environment but must rely on parents or carers to judge the correct heat of his room, the number of blankets on his cot and what clothes he should wear. Controlling children's environment is such an important part of caring for their health that it is essential that all aspects of the subject are clearly understood.

A Barrage of Infection

During the first few years of a child's life, infinitely more demands are placed upon his systems than they were originally designed to tackle under primitive conditions. From a very early age we are subjected to much more airborne infection than nature intended. In primitive days man would have wandered about in small groups and, as in

other natural herds or packs, there was probably no inter-
change between groups. There would be few young
children and thus the minimum of contact with new infection. Nowadays babies go about in prams and are admired
by an endless stream of people. Then there are shops,
supermarkets, playgroups, parties, bus rides, holidays –
all a possible source of new infection. Hardly a day goes
by when a child is not close to another child or a strange
adult who may well pass on a bug through a touch, a
cough or a sneeze.

From the moment a child is born huge demands are
placed on the lymph system. A newborn has not come
into contact with any infection at all so the lymph system
must work hard to fight every bug that he comes across
and produce antibodies for future protection. A small baby
has a huge lymph system in comparison to his tiny body.
However, the lymph nodes are very small compared to
those of an adult and unfortunately the bacteria, viruses
and dead cells are all full-sized. It is thus considerably
easier for the lymph nodes of the very young to become
overloaded.

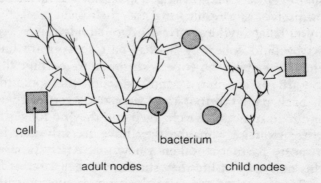

cell

bacterium

adult nodes   child nodes

Figure 4

Lack of Exercise

In all but professional sportsmen, our present lifestyle is sedentary compared to primitive days when we would have been continually on the move. As we have seen, the heart pumps blood out to all parts of the body. However, by the time it reaches the capillaries the blood is at almost zero pressure and depends to a great extent on the force of the muscle pump to return it to the heart. It is for this reason that we are designed to spend most of our time in moving our muscles and thus activating the muscle pump – if you watch a troop of chimpanzees or gorillas, for example, they are constantly on the move.

When you spend a lot of time sitting, standing or only walking then the muscle pump receives little activation and although the body's requirements are less, there is still not an adequate return of blood back to the heart. As a result of the poor circulation, excess fluid and waste products start piling up in the tissue spaces. It's very important that you take time each day to get all your muscles moving in order to boost tissue circulation. Everyone who does regular exercises acknowledges that they feel a lot better in themselves as a result.

If you have anything wrong in your body this is aggravated by fluid collecting in that part so you are undermining your ability to cope with the more chronic illness if you are too sedentary. Many patients who come to me with back pain say that they were once very active but their circumstances have changed and they no longer have time for exercise – maybe they have recently married a non-sporty partner or taken a new job. After six months of this new way of life they suddenly suffer a lot of back pain. This is due to the sluggish tissue circulation causing a gradual build up of waste products in the tissue spaces.

Exercise produces a large quantity of heat so it has

always had the benefit of keeping you warm without resorting to extra layers of clothing. If you have been sitting still for a long period of time you will feel much colder than someone who has been on the move.

Over-clothing

In children, it is the lymph system of the throat and lungs that is most commonly impaired. The rest of the system is rarely challenged until later in life. To explain why children are so vulnerable to constant colds and throat infections and to enable parents to take an active part in their child's health care, it is necessary to look at the way the body reacts to changes in its environment especially the temperature.

One of the biggest single advances that the human body has made was to shed its fur. One design difficulty with all engines is to provide for an adequate cooling device to dispose of the waste heat that is always generated. Animals have solved the problem of dissipating the considerable heat generated by muscular activity by 'panting' air. They have a very large blood supply to their nose and throat, and the action of 'panting' immediately cools down this very vascular area and so also cools the blood and body as a whole.

Man, however, developed such efficient muscles for his weight that this mechanism was not adequate, especially for the more prolonged effort that a human is capable of sustaining. Whereas a cheetah's muscles may give out at the end of a comparatively short run forcing it to stop 100 feet from its target, humans can endure a marathon. We are the only animal capable of such sustained effort and to achieve this we had to develop a new cooling system.

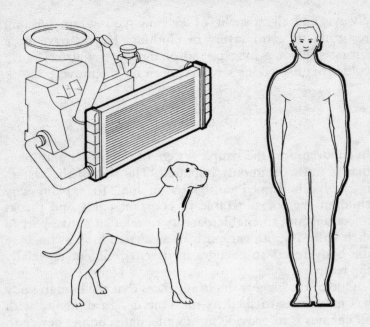

Figure 5: Illustration shows heat radiation (hatched areas).

By shedding our fur, humans increased the radiating surface from that of the tongue and throat to the whole body area. We also increased the cooling effect still further by sweating to evaporate fluid. (Small babies, who may be somewhat vulnerable to cold temperatures, are provided with a thick layer of fat to insulate them from loss of heat, including around the hands and feet. As they become older and start to run round, thus generating more heat, they lose this fat – the chubby baby vanishes to be replaced by a slim little child.) This means that humans, by varying the amount of blood and sweat to the skin, are able to maintain a constant body temperature over a wide variation both of the external heat and of muscular effort.

If the mechanism were allowed to develop fully of its

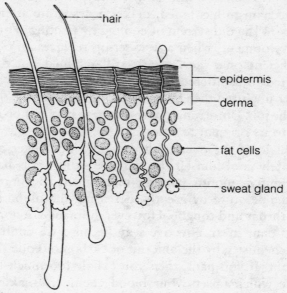

hair

epidermis

derma

fat cells

sweat gland

Figure 6

own accord, then we would need no clothes to maintain a normal body temperature under practically all conditions. There is the true story of a Sherpa, who, dressed in his loin cloth in an expedition well above the snow line in the Himalayas, was offered a suit of clothing on the grounds that he must be feeling the cold. Refusing it he protested, 'Me not feel the cold, Sahib. You see, me FACE all over.' The very small have not developed an adequate body temperature control but clearly even babies require help only with extremes of temperature otherwise the human race could not have survived.

As soon as we start putting 'fur' back on our children with lots of clothing, fleece-lined body suits and warm blankets then their bodies are no longer able to cool down in the way that nature intended. Instead such children are likely to become too hot. So the body, since its skin radiator mechanism has failed, makes a desperate attempt to go back to the old system of cooling by panting. Throughout development, when a new set-up replaces an older or less efficient one, the latter is still retained but may be converted to a different use. If the new system is demolished or impaired then nature tries to reinstate the old one to do the job. Unfortunately, this system may not be able to revert to its original function.

In this case the over-clothed child – no longer able to adequately cool himself through the skin – falls back on the primitive mouth panting mechanism to control his body temperature by greatly increasing the blood supply to the throat and tongue. However, humans are no longer able to pant in an effective way because we control our blood chemistry by the amount of carbon dioxide that we blow out. If you pant, then you exhale too much carbon dioxide which upsets your blood chemistry making you feel faint. You could even lose consciousness. As we can no longer pant a large quantity of air, the excessive fluid in the throat which comes from the increased circulation is not evaporated, resulting in congestion in the membranes of the nose and throat. This leads to a reduced resistance to bacteria and viruses, the lymph nodes become overloaded and the whole lymph system is less able to cope. The child succumbs more easily to infection and then finds it harder to fight it.

My daughter, Amanda, was only lightly clothed at any time. One cold Christmas afternoon when she was four years old we treated her to visit the London Zoo. Despite the snow on the ground, she was wearing a cotton shirt and a brief skirt, cotton socks and shoes and she was happily hopping and skipping all over the place, looking at everything that interested her.

We noticed another child in the zoo, trailing behind his parents, zipped into a wool-lined suit with his face just sticking out of the hood. My wife remarked that she felt really mean, as this other child looked much more cosy and warm than our daughter; but I pointed out that Amanda was infinitely more lively and active. I also commented that I suspected that the over-clothed boy was probably never well. My wife replied that it was easy for me to say that as we would never actually know the truth.

By a strange coincidence, about six months later we were invited to a dinner part in Hampstead. My wife immediately recognized one of the other guests, and during pre-prandial drinks, went up to her with a view as to where they had met. After some discussion she finally worked out that the fellow guests were the parents of the child we met at the zoo. Sure enough, the boy was very sickly and spent a great deal of time in hospital with constant attacks of bronchitis and pneumonia. Her parents said that it was so worrying because nobody seemed able to pinpoint why he was getting so many infections. He had always been a sickly child and they looked after him so carefully and gave him the finest food and vitamins, that it seemed unfair that he was never well.

It is always with the best intentions that parents over-dress children, but in the interests of your child's health it is important to supress your natural instinct to keep him warm and cosy. Children actually hate being too warm. There are so many occasions when I see a child yelling as mother insists on wrapping yet another blanket on the pram, and then kicking in an attempt to displace the offending covering. As soon as the little person succeeds, the blankets are immediately replaced, sometimes to the accompaniment of a howl of rage.

People often tell me that their children cry at night and no reason can be found. This is usually because they are too hot. Such children are nearly always sweaty and trying desperately to get rid of their bed clothes. The answer is simply to remove some of the covers. When clothing is kept to a minimum then the child is happier and the crying stops. Humans need to be able to cool down through their skin by sweating – if every inch is covered with layers of clothing then this natural mechanism is hindered and the child suffers greatly. I shall never forget visiting one such child in his nursery at home.

George's parents phoned to see if I would come to the house to see him. They said that he was only 18 months and had such bad asthma that he was too ill to travel. After hearing the story I agreed that I would go out and see him. He was having very bad attacks of asthma and his parents used an oxygen cylinder when the attacks seemed life-threatening. George had been in hospital twice already.

When I arrived at the house I was shown to the nursery. Although it was late spring, I was hit by a wall of heat as I walked through the door. The nanny took me over to the cot and there on top was a fur eiderdown. Underneath that was a quilt and then three blankets and a sheet. Under this was a bundle of clothing several layers thick, which once removed, finally revealed little George. He was absolutely soaking wet with sweat and had a rash on his neck and bottom.

A 'rattle' in his chest could be heard; the lymph nodes in his neck were already enlarged. There was also a tight feel to the muscles at the root of the lung. I tactfully explained to his mother that man had shed his fur to enable us to lose heat. By somewhat overdoing the 'putting back the fur' on George, the membranes of his nose and throat had become so swollen that fluid was actually pouring from them down to the lungs. I told her that as so young a child was largely unable to cough the mucus out, he tried to prevent the fluid from entering the lungs by the tubes closing down in a spasm. I suggested that if she slowly started reducing the clothing and heat in the nursery and let some fresh air into the room, then she would be going a long way to helping make her son better again.

She understood what I was telling her and three weeks later she rang to say that George was so much better and did she really need to bring him for treatment? Remembering the enlarged lymph nodes I suggested that she did bring him so that I could check that everything was alright. He needed three treatments on the lymph nodes but remained fit from then on.

Mothers often ask for guidelines for the correct amount of clothing, but it is very difficult to give any as every child has such differing requirements. A plumper child probably loses less heat, but then a thinner child is probably more active and generates more heat. When out of doors, my guide is: try to let your child do without a coat, even in winter. Carry a coat, or a pullover, with you, just in case your child tells you he is cold. Children are far more likely to be upset by being over-clothed than being too cold. If they are cold then they will let you know, either by yelling or, if the child is old enough, by asking. Instead of saying, 'You must put on your coat', try 'You should be warm enough but I have a coat if you need it'. You may well be surprised at how little your child actually needs in the way of clothing when he is running around outside.

To test for temperature in a very small person place a finger down the back of your child's neck. If it is warm, then your child is warm enough. There is no point in feeling hands and feet as nature doesn't waste energy in keeping hands and feet warm when so much is needed for growing, playing and learning. In the very young, Nature conveniently puts a thick layer of fat on fingers and feet – making them appealingly chubby – to insulate the inner person from the outside cold. If your child has very warm hands or feet then it means that the heat has got through all the fat insulation to the outside and the child will be grossly overheated.

There is a large degree of habit about your reaction to temperature; so it is wise to start teaching good habits at a young age. Temperature is relative – if you always want too many clothes then you get to the point where you feel very cold if you take your coat off whereas another person standing beside you could feel quite hot. There's a very interesting experiment to illustrate this point – take one bowl of iced water and one bowl of hot water. Put one hand in each and leave them for about 30 seconds. Now put them both in a third bowl of tepid water. Your hands will give out two different messages about the same water – to one, the tepid water seems unbearably hot; to the other, it will be very cold.

Positive Ionization and Pollution

Another factor which can weaken the lymph system is over-exposure to positively charged ions in the air. It's a stock joke with doctors that when people come home from a really healthy skiing holiday in the mountains with clean air, snow and sunshine, they catch flu on the plane or during the first few days back. This is directly related to the charge of the ions in the air. In a country such as Switzerland there are few bacteria or dust particles and those that are present are charged with negative ions. The body does not react to negative ions in the atmosphere and so its defence mechanism is not challenged and more or less switches off. On return to England, the body is not at all prepared for the instant attack of a bug, maybe passed by a sneeze on the aeroplane, and it is not difficult

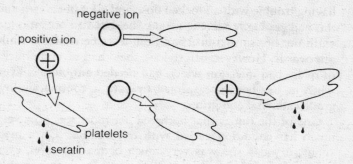

Figure 7

to understand that people succumb to an infection easily. In this country, with our heated homes and pollution, the air we inhale tends to be charged with positive ions. The body reacts badly to positively charged particles. If you breathe them in they pass through the walls of the lungs into the blood and affect the platelets causing them to produce excess quantities of a substance called serotonin. Although this is an important chemical messenger in the body, if too much is produced then it has undesirable effects. Excessive serotonin causes a swelling or inflammation present in the body greatly to increase. This will thus increase the congestion around the nose and throat area, particularly in young children, and so aggravate any infection already present; or make you more liable to catch another one.

The direct effect of positive ionization on health is well illustrated by one of my patients, 58-year-old Gladys, who noticed how her catarrhal condition changed with the weather. When the air was charged with positive ions her condition was dramatically worse.

Gladys had been catarrhal as a child and had always caught colds rather easily. By the time she was 30 she started having trouble with a blocked nose and a lot of catarrh and this had gradually become worse. She'd had an operation to wash out her sinuses and had been a lot better for a while afterwards. However, before long she'd had several attacks of really bad infection which had needed antibiotics. Even when at her best, she seemed to have a continuous low grade catarrhal condition.

One of the things that bothered her most was how very much her condition varied with the weather. On a nice, sunny, dry day she was very much better. However, even before the clouds started rolling in, her catarrh would gradually get worse. She could actually predict in advance when the weather was going to break or improve by the way that she felt.

She had also noticed that quite often, especially in summer and autumn, the weather preceding a full moon was good and she felt well. Just about the time of the full moon, the weather tended to suddenly turn and she would become very bad indeed. The other thing she had noticed was how bad she felt during the build up to a thunderstorm. As soon as the storm broke and there were a few flashes of lightening to negatively charge the particles in the air around her, her condition would improve enormously.

Stale air is charged with excessive positive ions which can greatly diminish the body's ability to cope with everyday bugs. As we breathe out, we increase these positive ions, so it is important to have plenty of fresh air to remove them and replace them with negative ions. If you live in a house where the windows and doors are kept firmly shut and no draughts are allowed in then the atmosphere is constantly charged with positive ions. We all need contact with fresh air, especially children who should be encouraged to play outside to get the full benefit of it.

Stale air is often associated with warmed air. All forms

of heating give out positive ions. With open fires these ions are pulled up the chimney so do not affect the atmosphere. However, other heaters tend to have a detrimental effect on the air in the room, depending on the degree of turbulence. A fan heater produces a large number of positive ions and most of us known instinctively that it is an uncomfortable form of heating. Even worse are the effects of air conditioning. Circulating fans cause turbulence and as air passes down ducts it tends to become more positively charged. In modern buildings where space is at a premium, ducts tend to be smaller and the air flows through them faster. This markedly increases the rate of positive ionization and is probably the cause of the 'sick building syndrome' in office blocks. Artificial heating, or air conditioning, is not a good environment for anyone to live or work in and is certainly not healthy for children. It is unnecessary to have any form of heating in a bedroom.

There is no doubt that pollution can further exaggerate the problem. A number of the substances involved in urban pollution are irritating in themselves, e.g. smoke, grit, dust, soot from exhausts of engines (especially diesels) and factory smoke. There are also gases such as sulphur dioxide and carbon disulphide, aldehydes and hydro-carbons. Pollution diminishes the actinic rays of the sun preventing the restoration of negative ionization. This results in the polluting particles being even more irritating. When a membrane is swollen it becomes sticky and the little hairs on the surface which move in organized waves to push specks up off it become completely engulfed in the swelling. When this happens, irritating particles can land and fix on the membrane and then inflame it. The membrane becomes swollen, blood rushes into the area, and this increases the congestion. The membrane tries to wash away the irritating particles or gases with secretions which

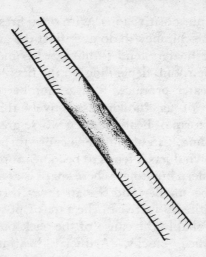

Figure 8

flow out, causing a discharge. Finally, the membrane itself swells so much that it can obstruct passages.

My treatment will reduce the adverse effects of pollution by restoring the normal function of the membrane. A negative ionizer will help diminish the irritating effect of any particles in the air. Most machines take more than an hour to modify the ions in an average room, which is not satisfactory, since normal ventilation changes the air several times an hour. The ionizer can never catch up.

Lack of Use

A lymph system can also be weakened by lack of use – either by being shielded from all contact with other people who may be carrying an infection, or by extreme caution over the food and drink that is consumed. Everything in the body is as strong as the requirement we put upon it. We have said in previous chapters: it contains a great deal of machinery in a small space. As part of the space saving project, the body only maintains and develops those systems that you are actually using. If you were to put your arm in a sling for long enough then you would gradually lose all your muscles there and eventually it would be completely useless. You have to use everything in your body to keep it going. The lymph system is no exception.

There is no doubt that frequent attacks of infection everyday are needed to maintain a vigorous defence mechanism. If older children, who have acquired most of their immunities, are protected from all infection then they tend to be the very ones that seem to 'go down with everything' as they have poor immune systems and do not cope so well. Clearly there are certain diseases where you are better to have some protection, such as measles, mumps, German measles, infantile paralysis and tuberculosis, but, as a general rule, it is not wise to guard your child from the run-of-the-mill infections.

In the same way, it is important not to be over-cautious about bacteria in the food and drink we consume. Under primitive conditions, humans were scavengers as well as hunters and would eat almost anything. If they came across something that had been killed by another animal then they would probably eat it – bugs and all. In order to cope with this stream of bacteria we developed a very effective defence mechanism with many circulating antibodies manufactured in advance. Although basically completely specific, antibodies can also have a more general, but weaker, effect on other bacteria of the same group. Clearly, the more antibodies you have, the more chance that one will be able to attack the bacteria immediately, even before your body begins to produce the specific antibody against that particular invader, which may take two or three days.

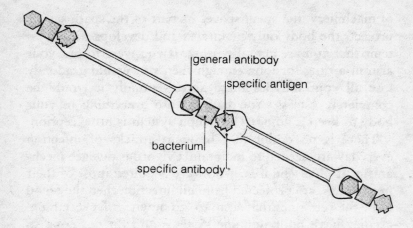

general antibody

specific antigen

bacterium

specific antibody

Figure 9

These days we seem to use all methods possible to decrease the number of bacteria coming into contact with our systems. For example, food is sterilized and kept in fridges both in shops and at home; sell-by dates are imposed; additives are put in to prevent bacteria and fungi from growing; food is deep-frozen, often after sterilization; fruit, vegetables and meat are stored in shrink wrappings, or protected in other ways, from the flies and wasps that would have been all over them fifty years ago. In my view, all these measures are basically wrong. 'Sell-by' and 'use-by' dates are a brilliant invention of food manufacturers to legitimize the waste of huge quantities of perfectly usable food. How many third world countries would give anything to obtain a share of these rejects? Years ago, my boys were having a party with a number of friends, so my wife left them some delicacies to eat at some time in the evening. The horror film finished at about ten minutes past midnight; it was time to eat! Someone inspected the 'use by' date and it had expired at midnight – no-one would touch the food. How do we reconcile this with eating game that has almost fallen off the hook? Yoghurt is milk gone bad, blue cheese is milk gone bad, gone bad, the list is endless. Even beer is malt, and wine grapes, gone bad. A strange convention excepts some foods from the 'gone bad' ban. Few housewives are unable to tell if a food is over the top, and this would be long after the sell-by date. By reducing the bacteria in our food and drink we are reducing the power of the reticulo-endothelial system (that part of the lymph, spleen and bone marrow system involved in the production of red cells, white cells and antibodies) to produce antibodies. This makes our immediate response to infection less effective and also reduces the number of circulating antibodies and thus our overall resistance. It used to be very very rare for anyone to catch a harmful bacterium from food. If they did, their defense mechanism was strong so the effect was minimal – far less than the mildest bacteria cause today. People now are always going down with one 'tummy bug' or other – in my youth these infections were unknown.

In the days when I went shopping with my mother the meat and fish would be left out on marble slabs covered with flies. Fruit and vegetables would be blanketed with wasps. Insects were very difficult to deal with in the home and kitchen and tended to climb over most of the food. Our bodies were used to dealing with a daily onslaught of bugs and we had so many circulating antibodies that when infections came along most of them didn't stand a chance.

Obviously, babies are very susceptible to infections until they have a chance to develop some immunities so a high level of sterility is important, particularly with the equipment they use for feeding and drinking. In primitive days, young babies would have been fed with breast milk, which is of course completely sterile, until an age when they had developed sufficient antibodies to cope with invaders and I firmly believe that breast milk is the best food for babies.

All this does not mean that personal hygiene is not important. Infections and infestations can be passed from the excreta to other humans and, being specialized invaders, can have very unpleasant effects. Washing one's hands after visiting the toilet is of paramount importance. Washing before preparing food is also a 'must'.

Dormant Trouble

Many children have very strong lymph systems and, despite modern conditions, cope with infections in their early years remarkably well. By the age of six or so they have a wide range of circulating antibodies and are able to fight common infections without any obvious breakdown in their lymph system. However, there are many other children who have somewhat weaker lymph systems, which may be a hereditary trait or the result of an acute infection such as flu early in life or the impact of our modern lifestyle. These children have a miserable first few years with a constant stream of sore throats, colds and other ailments.

These children who have a poorly start to life may appear to 'grow out' of all their problems by around seven years of age – and the early setbacks are all but forgotten as parents breathe a huge sigh of relief. However, although the problems may appear to be over, these children have often not fully recovered; the underlying trouble still remains. They have simply got to a stage where, thanks to the combination of their store of immunities and the efficiency of other defence mechanisms within the body, they can tolerate everyday infection.

The lymph system has actually been given such a battering that it may never fully recover without treatment both to clear the lymph nodes and stimulate the repair mechanism. By the time these children reach their mid twenties, and their natural repair systems start to slow down, it is quite common for them to start having problems again; often starting after a particularly virulent infection such as flu.

I saw Josh, 29, because he was having sinus trouble and bronchitis. He explained that as a child he had suffered from a large number of colds and sore throats. This had gradually improved as he became older and by the time he was eight years old he seemed to have got over the weakness and was quite well.

When he was 24 he had a bad attack of flu accompanied by sinus trouble and bronchitis. The flu took its course but he was left with painful sinuses and a tendency to bronchitis. When I saw him he was still catching frequent infections which went straight to his chest. He had been given various courses of antibiotics but the trouble had always returned.

On examination, he had a number of enlarged, hard lymph nodes that could be felt in his neck. I diagnosed that these had become partially blocked by the infections in his youth and that as soon as he had got all his immunities and with the resilience of youth on his side he had made an apparent recovery. However, the flu had overloaded his still defective defence system and reactivated the problem caused by the blocked nodes. Treatment with physical medicine to unblock the nodes and restore proper drainage from the sinus, throat and bronchial membranes stopped further attacks.

A lymph system, such as Josh's, that has been overloaded in its early years does not fully recover without appropriate treatment. Similarly, systems that have become partially blocked later in life through a series of low-grade infections, or one or two acute infections, will not function properly until proper lymph drainage is restored. In the following chapters we will look at the problems related to a poor lymph system. Chapter 3 looks at diseases associated with damaged tonsils, adenoids and the appendix. Chapter 4 looks at how blockage of the cervical nodes can lead to diseases including sinusitis, middle ear infections and loss of voice. Chapter 5 examines the thoracic lymph nodes and their association with bronchitis, asthma and related breathing problems. Chapter 6 shows how partial blockage of the abdominal lymph nodes can give rise to cystitis, painful periods and polyps and in Chapter 7, we study diseases associated with the inguinal lymph nodes, such as an arthritic knee, athlete's foot and leg ulcers.

3

THE FIRST LINE OF DEFENCE
UNDER FIRE

Everybody knows the name of the tonsils, adenoids and appendix, but how many people actually know what can go wrong with them and what ought to be done about it?

In their position at the front end of the lymph system the tonsils, adenoids and appendix are in the direct line of fire and are the first protective mechanisms to fight infection in the throat (tonsils and adenoids) or bowel (appendix). If the walls of these strongholds are attacked and eventually broken down this may cause a series of related problems. Unfortunately, there is an element of confusion surrounding these important specialized lymph nodes so this chapter aims to give a clear idea of the facts.

The Tonsils

Tonsils are frequently attacked by bacteria in the mouth, which we breathe in and take in on food, and also by those that come down from the nose. As we have seen in the Author's Note, healthy tonsils are capable of dealing with a wide variety of different infections. However, a point may be reached where tonsils, especially those that are inherently weak or those that have been weakened by previous damage, cannot cope any longer. Tonsils may be attacked by a number of separate infections which gradu-

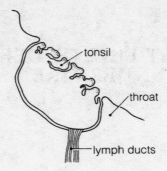

Figure 10

ally fill them with debris so that their channels become partly blocked. Bacteria are now not so easily dealt with by the impaired tonsils and eventually are able to break through the membrane of the crypt into the tonsils themselves and damage the mechanism. Sometimes they can be attacked by a single infection from a very powerful bacterium, which can largely overwhelm them, most commonly the β *haemolytic streptococcus* (Greek: *haima*=blood: *lysein*=loosen; so, red cell destroying, releasing the haemoglobin; *streptos*=curved: *kokkos*=berry; because it looks like a curved string of berries).

The Legacy of Damaged Tonsils

If damaged tonsils are not removed then they can cause prolonged ill-health at best, or serious illness at worst. Although symptoms other than a sore throat may not always be present at an early age, they can arise later in life. Conditions associated with damaged tonsils include:

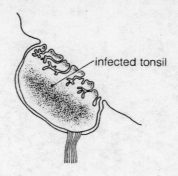

infected tonsil

Figure 11

RECURRENT TONSILLITIS, SORE THROATS AND OTHER INFECTIONS

When a healthy tonsil is working to fight an infection, the lymph drains from it into the tonsil node which is just below the angle of the jaw. If the tonsil comes under pressure from the infection at first this lymph node will help out the tonsil, but eventually it also becomes cluttered with the debris. The drainage of lymph through the obstructed node diminishes, further embarrassing the tonsils. In such a situation, the tonsils can no longer defend themselves adequately against the bacteria attacking from outside. So the bacteria are able to storm through the walls of the crypts and invade and damage the structure of the tonsil itself.

The tonsils have the special function of taking bacteria and viruses into their crypts and then producing antibodies against them. If the tonsils are damaged, they cannot produce these antibodies, so they are less able to fight the invading bacteria. The blood supply to the damaged tonsil is minimal and therefore any antibiotic has little or no effect on these bugs.

The tonsils become, in effect, a comfortable rest home

63

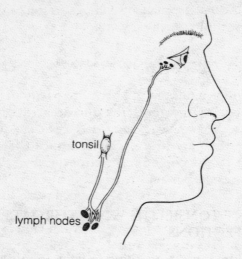

tonsil

lymph nodes

Figure 12

for tired bacteria to recuperate and multiply so they can launch a further attack on the throat. They have become a pool of infection which cannot be resolved and thus provides a constant source of re-infection to the throat. The longer the situation lasts, the more damage occurs to the lymph drainage of the throat area, the attacks become even more virulent and frequent and become harder to shake off.

Tonsillitis will usually clear up on its own in three or four days. It is not advisable to give antibiotics every time someone has a sore throat. In fact, quite the reverse. People should be allowed to acquire immunities to the various bacteria so that the chance of catching these infections again becomes steadily less. If a person has a really sharp sore throat, this is probably a strep throat which is usually accompanied by a fairly high temperature and the person feels definitely unwell. In this case the doctor will give an antibiotic at a fairly early stage, because this particular

infection can cause permanent damage to the tonsils, ultimately necessitating their removal.

CATARRHAL SECRETIONS

When the lymph nodes in the neck are partly obstructed,
the congestion in the nose and throat area causes the
membranes to become waterlogged as this extra fluid now
has nowhere to drain. Mucus glands in the affected membranes react to the potential infection (and irritations in
the air) by secreting mucus to wash it away. This mucus
first appears in the nose and throat giving rise to a runny
nose and cough. It may also drain down the trachea
(windpipe), especially at night, and actually infect the tube
resulting in bronchitis (see page 95). Or it can cause irritation which can lead to allergies and eventually even to
asthma (see page 103).

> Michael was 15 when he came to see me. He had been a
> healthy baby but by the time he was about two he began
> to catch a number of colds each year. Gradually he became
> more and more catarrhal until he was beginning to have a
> runny and blocked nose most of the time and his life was
> becoming pretty miserable. He then began to have a number
> of sore throats every year. Eventually at the age of eight he
> had his tonsils and adenoids removed.
>
> His general condition did improve a great deal after this
> but unfortunately Michael still had a blocked and runny
> nose and still seemed to catch a lot of colds. He had also
> started to develop sensitivities and seemed to have hay fever
> throughout the year. He had had skin sensitivity tests which
> showed that he was slightly allergic to a number of different
> substances. He had been put onto antihistamine drugs,
> which did dry up his nose for a while but then their effect
> slowly wore off. When he came to see me he was a little
> bit slow in his academic career, his concentration was poor

and he was rather naughty and tended to cheek the teachers. His short-term memory was poor and he lost his temper rather easily. On examination, his nose had very swollen membranes. In his mouth there was a certain amount of discharge coming behind the palate from the nose and sinus area but the tonsil beds were healthy. In his neck there was a large number of enlarged, hard lymph nodes which could be felt right down from behind the ear to the collar bone.

I diagnosed that the lymph nodes in his neck had become blocked by the constant infection of his tonsils and that the back pressure caused by this was making the membranes swollen. This lowered their resistance to infection. In addition, dusts and pollens were able to embed onto these sticky, swollen membranes. Normal membranes would be shiny with little hairs sticking out that all waved together to brush particles off the membrane. (See Figure 8) However, in Michael's case, the hairs were not able to do their job, the particles settled and he became very sensitive to them.

I advised his mother that he should have plenty of fresh fruit and vegetables and that he needed extra vitamins especially A and D (Cod Liver Oil or Halibut Liver Oil capsules) and Vitamin C tablets. I also said that he should have plenty of fresh air, reduced heating and wear only the minimum of clothing.

He had 11 treatments to restore a normal function to these lymph nodes, at the end of which his health had greatly improved. His personality changed somewhat and he was now able to concentrate. I was told later that his work and behaviour at school improved very considerably.

These catarrhal secretions can also run down into the stomach – often giving rise to a gastritis. As a result such children often have very poor appetites. In extreme cases the secretions can also drain through the bowel into the lymph nodes in the omentum (the apron lining the abdominal cavity). This can ultimately damage the appendix (see page 90). The inflammation of the stomach makes it sensitive to certain foods leading to food intolerances. This causes a reaction in the membranes of the nose, throat and sinuses. They swell even more, which produces more catarrh, and so the condition is self perpetuating.

POOR CONCENTRATION AND TIREDNESS

Someone with damaged tonsils may show certain behavioural characteristics that are caused by the fact that the tonsil nodes are part of a group of lymph nodes in the neck that also drains the brain. (See diagram, page 64) If the tonsil nodes are blocked then this causes back pressure which, as we have seen in the previous chapter, can affect drainage from other systems sharing the same drainage route; in this case, the brain. This cerebral oedema is like a very mild form of concussion, which is also oedema of the brain, and has the same sort of symptoms.

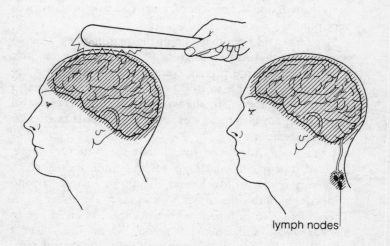

lymph nodes

Figure 13

67

Typical examples are children who do poorly at school and find it hard to mix with others. Teachers may criticize them for lack of concentration, poor short term memory and irritability, and give them a bad report. Parents find that the child is very often tired and objects strongly to being told what to do. These children make me feel very sorry for them as they are often punished for bad behaviour which they find impossible to control. It is quite remarkable how a child's personality can change once the damaged tonsils are removed and proper drainage from the brain is restored; as Anna's story testifies:

Anna was 11 when she came to see me. She'd had a number of catarrhal infections in her first two years of life. She then began to complain about ear-ache, and eventually had grommets put into her ears. This happened again two years later. Anna continued catching a number of sore throats each year and eventually she started to go a bit deaf. She had become exceedingly naughty at school and had even been thrown out of one school. Her academic progress was very poor.

Her father told me that one of the reasons they were so worried was that Anna was going to come into the majority of shares of a large private company when she grew up. Although he was able to stop her from getting these shares until she was about 30, she would in the end get control of the company and there was some fear as to its fate under her management.

I examined Anna and found that she had very large, infected tonsils. She had huge tonsil lymph nodes, which were very tender to touch, and a chain of enlarged lymph nodes down both sides of her neck as far as the collar bone. There were also problems with her ears. I referred her to an Ear, Nose and Throat surgeon, whose judgement I trusted, and he immediately removed them. One tonsil actually had an abscess in it.

Anna's health improved almost as soon as she woke up from the operation. She then had treatment to restore the drainage through the lymph nodes in her neck and it was very pleasing to see the improvement in every aspect of her health and behaviour. She had nine treatments in all at the end of which the lymph nodes could hardly be felt. She had also become a much nicer young lady. It was a story with a happy end, because, once she had finished her education, her father secured her a place in the family firm to learn all about the different aspects of it. At the age of 21 she went on the board and very soon took the firm over. Anna exhibited great administrative and commercial powers and the company prospered considerably under her management.

If a child displays this kind of behaviour pattern; or has an obvious change in personality, then there may be a number of physical causes. Obviously major disorders – such as a cerebral tumour will be readily diagnosed, but give catarrhal problems very serious consideration. It is quite amazing how much difference treatment can make and this can have a major effect on their future lives. I feel very strongly that teachers and parents should be made aware that these problems are often the real cause of bad behaviour.

I was at a dinner party some years ago when a friend asked when the school holidays started. At this point our hostess burst into tears and fled from the room. My host signalled me urgently with his eyes to follow her out. I went and asked her what was wrong. She replied that she was dreading her son Christopher's return from school. She said that he was a truly ghastly child – so difficult and rude. Apparently, Christopher, who was only nine years of age, was making her life utterly miserable and she hated the holidays.

I was really shocked at this outburst because I had known

Christopher for several years and he always struck me as a very pleasant and polite young man. I asked her a lot of questions and she told me that he used to be an easy child until he had a bad attack of flu followed by sore throats and tonsil trouble when he was five. Soon after that he had had another attack of flu. From then on he was always going down with sore throats and seemed very prone to infection. When about seven, Christopher began to become very difficult and uncooperative. This change was put down to the fact that he had gone to a boarding school too early and felt rejected.

I was not so sure that the problem was psychological, so I asked her to bring Christopher to see me during the school holidays. On examination, he had some nasty looking infected tonsils and his ears looked as though they had had a number of infections. He had some large tonsil lymph nodes and a chain of glands leading from them. I suggested that the behavioural problem could be cerebral congestion and that his tonsils should be removed. This was done and he came to have a few treatments on his lymph nodes. Within a few weeks Christopher's personality had changed back to his former helpful and willing self. He went on to do very well at school and university, and school holidays were no longer a nightmare for his mother.

ECZEMA AND INFANTILE ECZEMA

Eczema, especially infantile eczema, is often directly related to damaged tonsils. In order to understand the link we must remind ourselves that under natural conditions humans are an opportunist animal and our digestive system is designed to cope with meat. We would have lived on the meat that we caught ourselves or stole from some weaker creature. Failing that we might find something that had been abandoned by an already replete predator. As a last resort we could eat vegetation.

This is very probably the basic reason for the success of the Hay diet. If our digestive system is originally designed to deal with only one type of food at any one time, it may have some difficulty in coping with the mixed diet inflicted on it under modern conditions. With fit people, our belaboured enzymes and digestive system manage to cope very well and their predicament goes unnoticed by the indulgent host. If, however, the stresses of life or some illness have taken their toll, our systems may not be quite so able to manage. Then it is a help to separate out the various classes of food and eat only one type at a time which allows the struggling system to cope once more.

With our primitive scavenger lifestyle we would have had to cope with a great deal of bacteria in our mouth, as the food we obtained may well have been somewhat putrid. Worse still, our mouths or throats could easily be scratched by a bone or damaged in a fight. In order to provide strong protection against the assault by bacteria, there is a disproportionately large amount of lymphoid tissue in the mouth and throat area. This includes the tonsils and adenoids and the various numerous lymph deposits.

To overcome these defences and then take up residence in the damaged tonsils, the bacteria usually need more than their own strength. Several of them, most notably the *haemolytic streptococcus* and the *strep* (short for streptococcus) *viridans* (Latin: *vireos* = green; they produce green pus), are capable of excreting several toxins one of which is designed to devitalize the membranes of the throat in order to overcome the defences and make life easier for the bacteria. As we have seen, the throat and tonsils have a large collection of blood vessels so these toxins can rapidly pass into the bloodstream. Unfortunately, this toxin affects not only the throat membranes but also any elsewhere in the body closely related to it. This includes the skin and the membranes lining the joints. As the two conditions have a common origin, patients often come to me with both eczema and aching joints but the two disorders will be discussed separately.

If skin is irritated by the toxin it may develop a red, often slightly raised, map-like rash; usually on the neck and over the upper part of the chest. This is known as a strep rash. Some years ago, when the streptococci were either more potent, or our resistance less effective, this red rash could cover a large part of the body. With it came the high temperature usually associated with an acute strep infection coupled with the malaise, the disease was known as Scarlet Fever. These days we never see it. With most people the whole of their skin is devitalized but there are no obvious signs of this. It is only when patches of skin are irritated by being rubbed or exposed to cold air, that these areas break down causing a typical red rash usually with some spots scattered through the area. When there is no clear cause this is known as eczema (Greek: *ekzein* = to boil over) because there is no clear cause. If the cause is known, it then becomes known as a Dermatitis (Greek: *derma* = skin; – *itis* = something wrong e.g. detergent dermatitis). The thin skin on the inner side of joints is a common place to find eczema, especially as it has the added stress of the movement of the joint.

Clerise, aged 27, was sent to me by a skin specialist because she was having aches in her fingers, her right hip and slightly in the left knee. When I examined her there was not a great deal to be seen in the various joints except that the fingers were a little swollen. However, one of the problems that she was suffering from was a large, red, irritating area of skin from the lower part of the neck down over about half of her chest. Clerise had been having this treated with various creams and ointments for some months. In my opinion, the trouble with the joints was likely to have been a toxin from an infection and I examined her throat to find large unhealthy looking tonsils and large tonsil lymph nodes. A chain of these nodes went down almost to her collar bone. I asked an Ear, Nose and Throat surgeon to look at her tonsils and he decided that they needed removing fairly rapidly. This was done and she felt enormously better in herself. However, the eczema and joint pains still remained slightly. She then had some treatment partly in our surgery and partly by herself at home – massaging her lymph nodes. As these went down the final soreness in her throat went away and her eczema and the pains in her joints completely vanished.

While damaged tonsils is a common cause of eczema, in adults there may also be other factors involved. With babies and young children, however, a weakened lymph system is by far the most dominant reason. If a child is over-clothed, and thus overheated, the throat is more liable to infection. His skin is also likely to be permanently moist and sodden as the child secretes sweat in a desperate attempt to cool down, much the same as the skin becomes soggy under a plaster that has been left on for too long. Combine this condition with the effect of the strep toxin and you have the almost only cause of Infantile Eczema. This does, of course, also apply to adults.

Allergies, especially food sensitivities, increase the blood to the skin and so are a common trigger for eczema. Common foods that cause upsets are cow's milk (the next substance to require a government health warning in my opinion) and white flour. The treatment of infantile eczema is usually quite simple – take off as many of the child's clothes as is possible and ensure he gets plenty of fresh air. In all but extreme conditions, it is wise to cut out the heating in the bedroom, unless it is exceptionally cold, eliminate any foods that you suspect are causing sensitivities and, if the tonsils are damaged, they should be removed. Massage to the lymph nodes in the neck area, particularly those in the lower part near the collar bone, is also helpful.

Alistair was just over two and a half when he came to see me. He had bad eczema in his elbows and at the back of his knees and thighs. It was also on the bottom part of his stomach and behind his right ear. The rash looked very red and angry and had some nasty raw patches especially in the creases of his knees.

Alistair had started having eczema fairly early in life at about six months. At that stage it was only a small patch behind his knees; it only really became noticeable when he caught a cold. It became really bad when he was weaned at nine months old. At between 18 months and two years, it had spread to all the other areas.

The eczema varied from time to time but was never without the crinkled, red, map-like rash with sore patches and little scabs.

On examination, the skin lesions were typical of infantile eczema. Unfortunately, it was very itchy and his mother found it very hard to stop him from scratching. Alistair had large lymph nodes both in his groin and his armpits. His throat was rather red and his tonsils were very large and somewhat infected. He had a set of large lymph nodes in his neck extending down from the tonsil node. I considered his problem was partly due to the state of his throat which was brought about by over-clothing and advised his mother to take off as much of his clothing as possible while still keeping him warm. I assured her that children of that age feel the cold a great deal less than adults think. I also said that he would need some treatment to the lymph nodes in his neck as well as to the groin and armpits which she could do at home. I suggested that I should see him every couple of weeks to check how he was progressing. The other piece of advice was to try to cut out cow's milk as completely as possible for a while and see if this made any difference. When his mother brought him back for a check-up she said that she had been massaging the lymph nodes as I had shown her and that he seemed a lot happier now that he was wearing much less clothing. The eczema had shrunk considerably and did not look so angry. After another eight weeks it had largely disappeared. His mother went on treating him and we gave him some ultrasonic treatment on the remaining areas of eczema and on his throat. Eventually the eczema faded. However about a year later, his mother brought him back as there had been a recurrence when he had caught a bad cold. It was almost certain that a streptococcal infection had invaded his throat while it was weakened by the cold virus and the toxins from this had devitalized the skin causing the ezcema to come back. After treatment, the eczema again faded out; however he had another small recurrence after a few months and his mother told me that she had put him back onto cow's milk. He came off the milk and was fit. About two year's later he was able to tolerate cow's milk without any obvious problems.

JOINT PAIN

As discussed above, the toxins which are put out by bacteria to devitalize the lining of the throat can also affect the similar membrane lining the joints.

Cynthia came to see me at the age of 31. She was not feeling at all well in herself. She tired easily and her brain felt woolly. Her other worry was that she was beginning to get pains in some of her joints. Her left knee had started aching about three months ago and it was very uncomfort-able, especially when going down stairs. Cynthia had been fully investigated but nothing wrong had been found. She said that two of the fingers of her left hand were somewhat swollen and painful, also the digit finger of the right hand. Sometimes she had a slight ache in her left hip.

When I asked about sore throats Cynthia looked a bit confused because she did not see any obvious connection. However, she told me that she had started having an occasional sore throat when she was very young. These had increased in numbers until she was 18 when her condition had started to improve. By the time I saw her the sore throats were only occasional and usually started if she caught a cold. On examining her, I could not find much wrong with her actual joints – although they were swollen and slightly tender, they all had full movement. Her blood count was normal. However, her tonsils were large and very unhealthy. She had very large lymph nodes associated with the tonsils and a number of others could be felt on both sides of her neck. I decided that one of the main problems was that her tonsils were damaged and I asked an Ear, Nose and Throat surgeon to look at her. He agreed with my diagnosis and took out her tonsils which were apparently in a very bad state indeed. When her system had had time to recover after the operation, Cynthia felt much more lively and considerably less tired. Best of all, the problems with her joints disappeared.

RHEUMATOID ARTHRITIS

Thankfully, Cynthia was successfully treated at a fairly early stage but for some people the condition can become extremely serious. If you suddenly develop an allergy to the toxins then you may get the crippling disease rheumatoid arthritis which often strikes at around the age of 18.

Emma aged 27 was my secretary. She had been a little prone to throat trouble but not so bad as to interfered too much with her job. Then one day she asked me if I would look at her wrist because she thought that she must have sprained it. She showed me a rather swollen, hot, painful wrist. She could not remember how she had sprained it. I then looked at her other joints and found she also had a swollen and tender ankle and several swollen fingers. I asked if she had a sore throat at the time and she said she'd had one for about three days. Her tonsils were heavily infected. A blood test was positive for toxins that can affect joints and a culture of the bacteria proved it to be *strep viridans*. I insisted that she should be rushed to hospital to have her tonsils removed immediately. All her joints flared up directly after the operation and she had a great deal of pain but this settled down in a few weeks. She did actually still have times, over the next couple of years, when she had a slight pain in her wrist but the trouble gradually faded out.

I am quite sure that if her tonsils had been left in for many more months she would have suddenly gone into a full-blown rheumatoid arthritis. Then it would, most likely, have been too late to do anything. Taking her tonsils out would not have cured the trouble because she would have developed an allergy to the toxins. In that case the minute infection still present in her throat would have been enough to have maintained the arthritis.

I cannot emphasize too strongly that if tonsils are infected and pouring toxins into the whole body, then they should be removed. Imagine that a munitions factory has been badly damaged by an explosion and has then been taken over by a street-gang. Not only do the children terrorize the neighbourhood with muggings (sore throats) but worse – they find that the town water main runs under the factory. They dig down to it and inject noxious substances into it that will affect parts of the town miles away. The gang of children are in a no-go area to the police so the only cure would be a giant bulldozer to get rid of the whole factory. Similarly, in my view, the only cure for the tonsils is to remove them as soon as it is established that they are damaged.

Tonsillectomy (removal of tonsils)

A number of mothers say that they have been told that their children's tonsils, although damaged, should be left in. If your child has recurrent sore throats and seems to catch a lot of colds then you should ask the question 'why?'. Suggest to your doctor that your child has his tonsils taken out. If he disagrees, yet from what you have read you feel strongly that this is the best course of action, then insist that it is done. Don't be fobbed off with comments such as, 'he'll grow out of it'. The symptoms may subside but this doesn't necessarily mean that the lymphatic system is in full working order.

The effect of removing healthy tonsils is negligible as other lymphoid tissue will take over their functions if these are needed, whereas the consequences of leaving them in can be very serious. I see a number of patients every year in middle age who are suffering from arthritis, tiredness, ME and other problems which could have been avoided if the tonsils had been removed at an early age.

To recap, tonsils should be removed

- If they appear small and pale (which means they are destroyed and no longer serve any useful purpose) or if they are large AND infected and the patient shows some of these clinical signs:
- The tonsil lymph node (under the angle of the jaw) feels enlarged and tender (painful on pressure) virtually all the time.
- A history of sore throats and a tendency to catch whatever bug is doing the rounds.

- Marked behavioural characteristics including irritability, poor short term memory, tiredness, lack of concentration and a poor performance at school.

The tonsils are self-contained units in a capsule; joined to the body by a stalk containing the artery, veins, lymphatic ducts and connective tissue. If the tonsil is removed in childhood then it is a fairly simple operation – severing the stalk will enable the tonsil to be shelled out of its capsule quite cleanly. The stalk may need tying off, but may just seal itself off without a tie being necessary. This is a very minor operation called enucleation and causes the minimum of disturbance to the patient.

If, however, destroyed tonsils are left in for a number of years, the patient will most likely suffer sore throats, constant infections and excessive tiredness. There are also the other problems associated with damaged tonsils which have been discussed above. A further disadvantage of leaving in infected tonsils is that if the inflammation reaches the edge of the organ, as it usually will, it will cause the capsule itself to become inflamed and sticky so that the tonsils adhere to it. Blood vessels grow across this gap

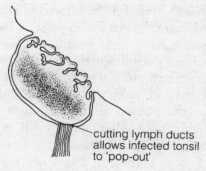

cutting lymph ducts allows infected tonsil to 'pop-out'

Figure 14: Long-standing infection of the tonsil.

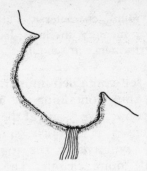

Figure 15: Enucleation of the tonsil.

and the tonsil slowly becomes merged with the surrounding tissues.

If the tonsils are removed at this later date the operation is an altogether more formidable undertaking. The tonsil will have to be cut out of the throat wall leaving a large raw area. Since there is no clear definition between the tonsil and the throat it is always possible that a little bit of the tonsil may be left in. This can jeopardize the outcome of the operation, and may itself need removal in the future. The post-operative recovery is obviously far less smooth than if the tonsil can be *enucleated*.

Even so, the discomfort after the operation is overwhelmingly worthwhile for the improvement of the throat itself and the general health of the patient. However, those sufferers who do have their tonsils out on the late side should be warned that although they may well feel enormously better immediately after the operation – almost as soon as they wake up from the anaesthetic – this may not last. Unfortunately, after about the tenth day, bacteria settle in the raw area where the tonsils were cut away causing a similar infection to the original one. The patient feels just as bad as before, and it is not until the normal protective throat membrane has grown over the whole area that the bacteria are finally thrown out. The patient will feel hugely better after about two months.

Mistaken Identity

Unfortunately it is sometimes the adenoids that are removed instead of the tonsils. This is often due to a misunderstanding of their role. When the tonsils are working inefficiently, the adenoids increase their workload to take over their job. As with all lymph nodes, the adenoids increase in size when they are working hard.

However, they have the mechanical disadvantage that the nasal passage around them is not very roomy so this enlargement can hinder breathing by blocking the passage of air from the nose into the throat. This is the reason, why all too often, healthy adenoids are the subject of the surgeon's knife and not the diseased tonsils.

Adrian, 14, was very catarrhal and blocked. He tended to breathe through his mouth. He said that he didn't feel very well, got tired easily and had poor concentration. Bad school reports confirmed this. He'd had his adenoids taken out when he was nine because of the respiratory obstruction; however this had only helped the breathing for a short time. Subsequently his overall condition seemed somewhat worse.

Like so many people with damaged tonsils, he had frequent sore throats and a tendency to catch lingering colds. When I examined him, I found that his throat was red and he had large, somewhat unhealthy looking tonsils. The tonsil lymph nodes were very large and very tender and there was a chain of enlarged lymph nodes leading from both tonsil nodes down his neck. This picture indicated that the tonsils were damaged and permanently infected and that the rest of the lymph nodes in the area were taking on an extra workload.

The adenoids had been removed in error. They were only enlarged because they were compensating for the damaged tonsils. Indeed they had become his main defence mechanism. By having them out Adrian had been left more vulnerable than ever to infection. Had his tonsils been taken out and his adenoids left in, then his adenoids would almost certainly have shrunk back to a normal size once they did not have to cope with the stream of infection from the tonsils. He would then have been left with a high resistance to infection and properly functioning lymph nodes.

Adrian required seven treatments to the nodes in his neck to clear the now semi-permanent blockage. After that he felt very fit and has remained so.

Damaged tonsils may be small and so be left in whilst the large, healthy adenoids are removed. The right thing is to take out the tonsils and let the surgeon carefully assess whether it is necessary to remove the adenoids as well. This can normally only be satisfactorily done at the time of the operation. Thankfully, the lymph system is very versatile so if you do destroy healthy adenoids then the body will regrow lymph tissue to take over.

The Appendix Vermiformis

In the same way that the tonsils are the first line of defence against infections of the nose and throat, so the appendix and large plates of lymph tissue called Peyers Patches protect the bowel wall. As the Peyers Patches only go wrong with very rare diseases, they are outside the scope of this book. The lymph system in the bowel is normally extremely powerful. However if the appendix is over-

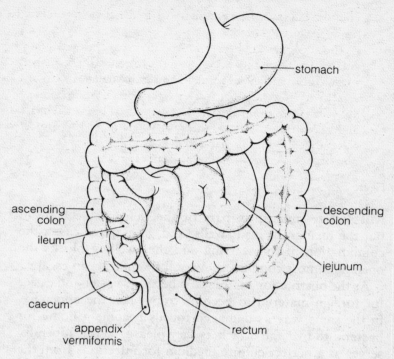

stomach

ascending colon

ileum

caecum

appendix vermiformis

descending colon

jejunum

rectum

Figure 16

loaded then the abdominal lymph nodes, into which it drains, may become blocked with the resulting debris. This gives rise to congestion and the appendix may become infected and inflamed.

At first these low-grade infections in the walls of the appendix are dealt with by the antibody response and the fighting white cells and there may well be no obvious symptoms. However, each attack leaves some more scarring in the wall of the appendix, usually half way along the tube, which progressively narrows the channel. This scarring does not go away so the narrowing is permanent. The mucus glands in the membranes lining the appendix

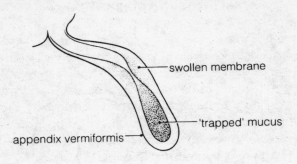

swollen membrane

'trapped' mucus

appendix vermiformis

Figure 17

will secrete mucus, as part of the defence mechanism, but the membrane also swells, and, in extreme cases, the combination of the scarring and the swelling blocks the opening almost completely. Very little mucus can escape.

As the obstruction increases, it becomes easier and easier for foreign material to become trapped in the appendix. In the same way as damaged tonsils become a home for bacteria to live and attack as they please, so the appendix serves as a perfect culture medium for infections from the bowel. The scarring means that the wall of the appendix is less able to defend itself, making it easier for the bacteria to invade the wall and then ultimately break through the appendix. Alternatively, the blocked-off part of the appendix can blow up as an abscess and this in turn can burst. In either case this leads to the very serious condition known as peritonitis (infection of the peritoneal membrane). In the days before modern treatment with antibiotics this condition was frequently fatal.

Chronic Appendicitis

Sadly, the early signs of a problem appendix are often missed and the condition can continue for some time, even several years, causing much distress. Often it is only diagnosed when it is too late and the condition has developed into acute appendicitis. Occasionally there are no symptoms associated with chronic appendicitis, but usually there are some warning signs which should indicate that there is something wrong.

STOMACH PAINS

When there is a low grade inflammation in the appendix wall in the early stages you feel pain about two inches above the umbilicus. You may think it strange that you should feel pain at this spot when the appendix is actually in the lower right quarter of the abdomen. To understand this, we need to consider how the nerve system works. Each little bit of skin has its own nerve endings which go to an indicator board in the brain. The indicators tell the brain which particular area is involved – so you are aware in which part of your body anything happens. If you touch your face, or your tummy, or your leg, then the brain registers which part has been touched. If your skin is damaged, or unreasonably stimulated, then you would feel pain there as the brain registers the part of the body that is affected.

However there are so many nerve endings it is not possible to have a separate indicator for every single one; so they have to share. And it makes sense that the sensors of the skin, which we use most, share with the rarely used ones of internal organs. In the case of the appendix – it has sensors in its wall, which are stimulated when there is local inflammation. However, the brain, thinks that these

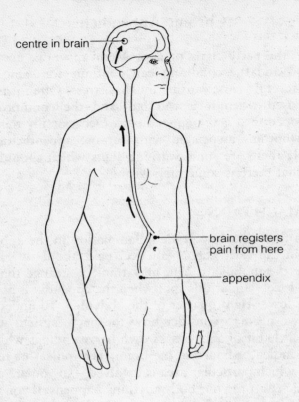

centre in brain

brain registers
pain from here

appendix

Figure 18

impulses are coming from the skin which shares the same nerve. After all, it is not possible for someone to pinch your appendix. So, when the appendix is inflamed the pain is felt about two inches above the tummy button, the site of the sharing skin.

If the infection breaks through the appendix and inflames the peritoneum, then the pain switches to the real site and is felt in the right, low side of the abdomen. This is because the peritoneum is so important that it has direct representation in the brain. If the tummy ache suddenly switches to a much sharper pain in the right side of the stomach this means that the infection is breaking through to the peritoneum and the child should be taken to hospital immediately.

My own daughter, Amanda, started complaining of nagging pains in her stomach when she was nearly two years old. We eventually took her to see a specialist at Great Ormond Street who explained that the pains were psychological. He said that Amanda was probably lonely as she was an only child and that some friends invited in to tea would help the problem. So we invited friends but it didn't help. We were told to invite friends for the whole day, the night, the weekend; but the pains continued.

Then about a year later we were on holiday playing on the beach, when she suddenly grabbed her stomach, burst into tears and went a waxy, white colour. This was the first time I had seen an attack but my wife said it was the same as the attacks she had been having all along. I immediately diagnosed appendicitis. We rushed Amanda home just too late. Her appendix had burst and she was desperately ill for some while.

PAINS IN THE BLADDER

Pain may also be felt in unexpected places such as the back or bladder or even in the knee. Women in particular often come to the doctor complaining of an irritable bladder, passing urine frequently and complaining about a condition that feels like cystitis. These symptoms arise because the inflamed appendix touches these parts of the body and also affects nearby nerves producing referred pain elsewhere. Due to the nature of the nerve system, the pain from an inflamed nerve is felt at the place the nerve supplies, not at the site of its stimulation.

I was getting up to go at the end of a play, when I suddenly got an agonizing pain in my right knee. I was 34 at the time. I was only just able to get home. I knew the trouble was not in my back or knee and the only thing I could think of was my appendix which occasionally touches the nerves that go down the leg. At three in the morning it was so painful that I asked my wife to telephone a surgeon immediately. 'My husband has acute appendicitis,' she said. When the surgeon asked how long the stomach pains had been going on, she replied, 'Oh, he hasn't got a pain in the tummy, it's in his knee!' When he heard this the surgeon was far from happy, but my wife insisted and he eventually agreed to see me at this early hour of the morning. Just as he was taking out my appendix, it burst, but fortunately it was removed in time.

GENERAL ILL HEALTH

Children, or indeed adults, with a chronic appendix are generally not well in themselves. Characteristic symptoms include:

- Tiredness almost all of the time. +
- Episodes of exhaustion for no apparent reason. +
- Poor appetite.
- Alternate constipation and diarrhoea.

In addition, there may also be sub-acute attacks of appendicitis with characteristic stomach pains accompanied by:

- Nausea.
- Greyness in face and a waxy white ring around the mouth. +
- A feeling of being threatened; a tendency to burst into tears. +

(+ These symptoms are caused by an upset of sympathetic/parasympathetic nerve relationship. If you wish to know more about this, it is fully covered in my earlier book, *The Back and Beyond* also published by Arrow Books).

These symptoms are often diagnosed as a condition called abdominal adenitis because it is thought they are caused by inflamed abdominal lymph nodes. However, I have always found this assumption rather unsatisfactory as lymph nodes are inert objects and they require to be inflamed by something. So if the abdominal lymph nodes are inflamed then it would be because of a catarrhal condition of the bowel. A common reason for this is that pus from the tonsils is swallowed and so upsets the bowel and appendix. The symptoms of abdominal adenitis are almost always cured by taking out the appendix.

A child may suffer from chronic appendicitis with subacute attacks for several years. Despite the fact that the child is obviously not thriving, a parent is often told that she will 'grow out of it'. Indeed, the symptoms may subside a little but the appendix is rather like a time-bomb just waiting to explode. When you feel the stomach of someone with a damaged appendix, the muscles in the lower right hand side of the abdomen will be tight. This condition, known as muscle rigidity, is nature's way of making a wall to protect the delicate appendix from the outside and is one of the classic signs that all is not well. When the appendix is removed under these conditions, it is usually found to be infected.

When Adam was about 9 he had a bad stomach upset which was diagnosed as a salmonella infection. This soon settled down but from then on he was never quite the same. He would get tummy upsets once or twice a year accompanied by cramp pains. He felt tired most of the time and had moments when he felt drained for no obvious reason. He had become a tiny bit tetchy and unreasonable but that was attributed to stress and worry at school. By the age of 14, he was still not on top form with occasional slight tummy upsets.

At 14, he had an episode of definite pain just above his tummy button. This was repeated the following year. Then suddenly, at the age of 17, the pain went down to the right lower part of his tummy and he started being sick and feverish. His mother recognized the signs of acute appendicitis and rushed him into hospital. As soon as his infected appendix was removed, Adam made a complete recovery and all these symptoms of the past disappeared.

If a damaged appendix is left in, then the underlying problem still remains and it only takes something like a change of food on holiday, or an attack of enteritis to trigger an acute appendicitis. The earlier that a damaged appendix is diagnosed, the sooner it can be removed before there is a serious health risk.

Causes of a Damaged Appendix

The main causes of damage to the appendix are: low-grade throat infections early in life; poor diet, especially too little roughage; and excessive amounts of laxatives, spicy foods and those to which the person has become sensitive. It would be helpful to look at these causes in more detail.

EARLY THROAT INFECTIONS

As we have seen, when children are subject to many throat infections then the tonsils may become overloaded. Phlegm and pus containing a lot of bacteria drain down from the tonsils to the stomach, bowel and possibly even the appendix. This infection may prove too much for an already over-worked appendix to cope with and it can no longer defend itself against attack.

Clara was 17 when she was brought to see me. She had had problems with her throat since she was about seven years of age. She'd had around two sore throats a year since then. From the age of about 12, she was beginning to become tired easily and was not concentrating well. She had also lost her appetite and become a faddy eater. At times she complained of vague pains in her tummy just above the umbilicus.

On examination, I found that Clara had large and heavily infected tonsils with enlarged, tender, tonsil nodes and she also had a certain amount of tightening of the muscles in the lower right part of her abdomen, where the appendix lies. This area was very tender.

My first action was to get Clara's tonsils removed as these were the most likely cause of the problem. After this, her general health improved somewhat – however, she still got tired very easily, and she had a white ring around her mouth and general paleness of colour, and the tummy pains continued. These signs all indicated to me that her appendix had become damaged and she was having episodes of sub-acute appendicitis. I consulted a surgeon who agreed to remove her appendix which was found to have been damaged. From then on Clara made a good recovery in every respect.

POOR DIET

Another cause of damage to the appendix can be a poor diet, especially one with too little roughage which can put the whole bowel under strain. The bowel moves the food we consume steadily down its length by a ring of bowel

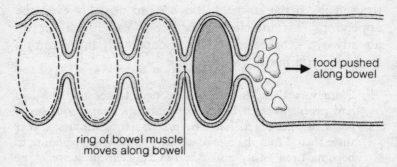

food pushed along bowel

ring of bowel muscle moves along bowel

Figure 19

muscle contracting so that the lumen is almost closed off. (See Figure 19.) This ring moves slowly along the bowel wall pushing the food in front of it. Much like the way a caterpillar moves around. If there is only a small amount of solids present this is not enough to stimulate your bowel movement properly; the solids can escape through the hole in the muscle ring and the waste is not propelled along as it should be. This can cause irritation, especially of the large bowel, as the larger hole would make the peristalsis (the pumping action of the bowel from the Greek: *perstellein* = to clasp) even less efficient.

Camilla, 37, wasn't feeling well and had a painful back particularly between the shoulders. These symptoms had been going on for about 15 years. She also got tired very easily and in the last few years was having trouble first of all with constipation and then an irritable bowel. She ate very little roughage so as not to upset her bowel but she was finding that she had to take laxatives almost every night to have any motion at all the next day. Her nails were brittle and cracked, she had very dry skin and her hair was thin and dull.

On examination, Camilla had an increase in her thoracic curve and her abdomen was tender, especially around the area of the large bowel. The membrane of her throat was red and swollen. There was some discharge in her nose. She had a number of enlarged lymph nodes in her neck on both sides and she also had a lot of oedema in the muscles at the root of the lung, a sign that there is trouble in the lymph nodes in that area. We decided that she had gastritis probably associated with the back problem and this had caused faulty absorption of vitamin B which largely accounted for her dry skin, cracked nails, straggly hair and possibly some of her tiredness. It was also clear that her bowel was having trouble with the inadequate amount of bulk so I put her on a high fibre diet and asked her to cut out milk as far as possible as I thought that it may have been causing a food sensitivity.

At first her bowels were exceedingly upset, so I put her onto a drug to soothe them down for a week or two. Gradually she came off the drug and, after a while, her bowels became more normal and she began to feel altogether better in herself. She did not need to have her appendix removed as the catarrhal state seemed to have made a good recovery.

As we have seen with the story of Camilla, lack of bulk in the diet can commonly cause constipation and also be partly responsible, along with food sensitivities, for an irritable bowel. Other associated problems include diverticulosis, where little balloons form as bulges in the bowel wall, usually at the site of muscle weakness where the blood vessels pass through them; and cancer of the bowel. Although lack of fibre is not the cause of bowel cancer, it is a fact that people who eat a high fibre diet have a significantly lower incidence.

EXCESSIVE LAXATIVES

While lack of bulk can cause problems with the bowel and adversely affect the appendix, excessive amounts of laxatives are also undesirable. So too are stimulating substances such as hot spices and any foods to which a person has become sensitive. All of these can hurry the digestive processs so the food arrives in the bowel partly digested. Bacteria can then infect the food, especially if there is already excessive fluid in the area which makes it very much easier for bacteria to spread around the bowel. Toxins from this bacterial activity can then mildly poison the muscles of the bowel wall causing some constipation. This situation makes it easier for the appendix bacteria to invade. Fortunately the stomach usually becomes acclimatized to foods such as curry, so these would cause only a temporary problem.

This chapter has dealt with problems with specialized lymph tissues; the next two chapters deal with the specific diseases that arise when groups of lymph nodes become obstructed.

4

A BREATH OF FRESH AIR

Bronchitis, Asthma and Other Breathing Problems

Over recent years the number of people suffering from asthma and the severity of the condition has increased at an alarming rate. In my early days as a doctor, asthma was not the life-threatening disease that it is today. In the light of such worrying statistics I find it rewarding to be able to reassure people that most asthmatic sufferers can be helped to enjoy an active life free from all drugs and sprays. One child who particularly stays in my mind is Bob, a patient at one of my hospitals. I first saw him at the age of five when he was so ill with asthma that he was going to be sent to a special school.

At the time, Bob was a very sickly boy who suffered badly with bronchitis and asthma. He had been in and out of hospital over the past two years and his condition was clearly getting worse. The doctors at the hospital were worried and asked if I might be able to help.

When I examined Bob, I found that he had huge lymph nodes in his neck and a tremendous spasm and swelling of the tissues in the middle of his thoracic spine, just where the root of the lung comes down. X-rays showed that the lymph nodes where the trachea divides into the two bronchi were indeed very waterlogged. I gave Bob treatment to the enlarged lymph nodes in his neck and thoracic region and arranged for him to have his unhealthy tonsils removed. After a couple of months, Bob's breathing problems started to improve quite dramatically and the attacks gradually became rare and very mild. He had an attack of asthma the following year when he caught a cold and then again two years later after a bout of flu. I gave him more treatment and heard nothing for a few years. Then one Christmas, his mother sent me a card asking if I remembered her asthmatic son. Well, not only had he been made head boy at a normal school, but he was also captain of the football and cricket team and was doing well academically.

Asthma is a curious disease which can be divided into two categories: allergic asthma, which is the true disease, and infective bronchitic asthma which is not actually a disease but a defence mechanism that has become so exaggerated it has become a disease. These two conditions are often confused and both labelled as asthma. However, it is essential to identify the particular type of asthma at an early stage so that the correct measures can be taken.

ALLERGIC ASTHMA

This, to my mind, is a comparatively rare condition and is not within the scope of this book. A few people have a serious allergy problem which can cause the bronchial tubes to close down when the substance involved is breathed in; however it is not common. When tests for allergies are performed on people with asthma, the majority have a number of mild sensitivities, whereas those performed on people with true allergic asthma result in one or two massive reactions to specific allergens such as cats, dogs, horses or pollens.

If you have true allergic asthma then you may be breathing perfectly normally one minute but, as soon as a cat comes into the room, you are fighting for breath. This is because your body recognizes the allergen that is being breathed in and however small the actual amount, it fears that there is going to be a massive influx so the whole of the bronchial tree goes into a protective spasm to try to keep the offending substance out. The onset is usually quite sudden and the disease does not come on step by step, as does the more common infective version.

Allergic asthma and hayfever are close cousins. As the membranes of the bronchial tree are more easily upset than those of the nose, a child tends to react to allergens first with asthma and then later in life, at around 15 or so, with hayfever.

INFECTIVE BRONCHITIC ASTHMA OR BRONCHITIS

Bronchos is the Greek word for a breathing tube – so bronchitis actually means an inflammation of the breathing tube. Although the symptoms of bronchitic asthma may appear to be somewhat similar to allergic asthma, they have very different causes. Bronchitic asthma is caused primarily by an infection. This can range from a constant infection caused by a low-grade bacterium which only just manages to infect the breathing tube, causing mucus to be secreted to wash the organism away; to a momentary virulent infection when the invaders of the breathing tubes cause them to become inflamed and produce in much mucus in much greater quantities.

Bronchitic asthma is a condition which is acquired as a response to the mucus in the breathing tube. It may involve the lower parts of the lung at first, as the mucus tends to drain into them. As it progresses, however, more and more of the lung may become involved until eventually the whole bronchial tree may go into spasm during an attack. This type of asthma is a defence mechanism which occurs particularly when the child is very small. Infection in the nose and throat causes secretion which runs down into the trachea. There is a risk that the mucus and debris caused by the infection may go into the lungs so, in order to prevent this, the bronchi go into a protective spasm to shut down the passages. In the very young this is essential because they have not learned to cough things out; so, if the lungs cannot expel something, it is supremely important to stop it from getting into them in the first place.

This defence mechanism can become so exaggerated that the effect of the spasm is a worse problem than the infection. Unfortunately, by the time that the child has learned to cough, the reflex or habit of the bronchial spasm has become firmly established and therefore persists into adolescent and adult life. This type of asthma is very much more common than allergic asthma. It will improve enormously from simple measures taken at home (see Chapter 1 and 2) and, if necessary in severe cases, by treatment such as I give in my practice; this is to restore the lymph drainage through the cervical and thoracic lymph nodes. However, for the treatment to be successful, the parents, or possibly the patient, must play a large part in the regime of recovery. It is therefore vital to be aware of the anatomy of the respiratory system and how a partial blockage of the thoracic lymph nodes can give rise to breathing problems.

Our Respiratory Tree

The thoracic lymph nodes are a large group of nodes which, as the diagram shows, are situated around the point where the two tubes, known as the bronchi, carry air between the trachea, or windpipe, and the lungs. The bronchi also run parallel to the lymph drains and the blood vessels coming in and out of the lungs; so, in effect, you have four trees going into or coming out of your lungs.

- The trachea, or windpipe, breaks up into the two bronchi, then into smaller and smaller bronchioles until they finally become the minute alveoli. These are the little sacks into which the smallest bronchioles join. The air in the alveoli contains a large quantity of oxygen which flows through the membranes lining them and into the blood where it is taken up by the red cells. Blood also contains a considerable amount of carbon dioxide as a result of metabolism (Greek: *metabole* = change; the chemical processes essential for life) and this flows in the reverse direction to be breathed out into the air. The oxygen actually pushes the carbon dioxide out of the blood. It is only in the alveoli that the gas exchange between the air and the blood takes place. The walls of the alveoli are folded in on themselves, rather like a three-dimensional three-leafed clover, to give the maximum possible contact between the gases and this surface area and so make the exchange as rapid and complete as possible. The exchange surface is so large that if you were to spread out flat all the alveoli from both lungs they would occupy the area of a full size tennis court with all its surrounds. The wall of each alveolus has an elaborate network of arteries, veins and lymphatics. With such a large area involved, it follows that there is an amazing number of blood vessels in contact with the air.
- The artery which carries in the stale purple/blue blood and forms a network all around the wall of each alveolus.
- The vein which carries the fresh oxygenated red blood back to the heart and so into the arteries supplying the body.
- The lymphatics which carry the fluid from the tissue spaces

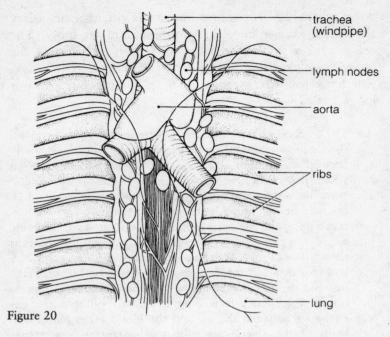

trachea (windpipe)

lymph nodes

aorta

ribs

lung

Figure 20

in the wall of the alveoli into the thoracic lymph nodes at the root of the lung. The lymph carries with it any particles such as dust and soot, bacteria or viruses which have been inhaled and any fluid which may have accidentally passed into the breathing tubes. The thoracic lymph nodes filter out the solids, producing antibodies against any infection present; they then get rid of the solids either by liquifying them, or letting the white scavenger cells engulf and carry them away. A huge system is needed to service the lungs as there is such a high risk of an attack by potential invaders.

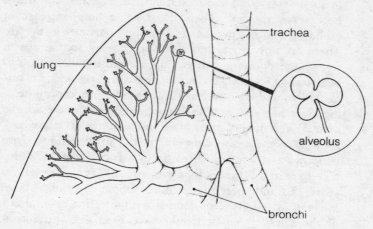

Figure 21

The Lymph Flow

The thoracic lymph nodes are positioned around and near the bronchi and any partial blockage is likely to have a major impact on the respiratory system. These nodes may become obstructed for several reasons:

- Throughout childhood the lymph nodes are relatively much the same size as the rest of the body so in a very small person they are very small. However, the particles in the air and invading bacteria are always the same size and therefore relatively much larger in a baby. It is all too easy for them to clog the lymph nodes of a child and, unless treated, this obstruction will continue to adulthood (See Figure 4).
- The lymph system was designed by natural selection to be adequate for the conditions in which humans evolved – unpolluted air, little or no clothing and restricted contact with only a few varieties of bacteria. As we have seen in Chapter 2, over recent years our lifestyles have changed

101

in such a way that the lymph system is almost certain to become overloaded. There has been a huge increase in pollution and the number of irritating particles in the air. There are now many more flowering trees and shrubs in streets and domestic gardens, all of whose pollens tend to be irritating – certain crops like rape also have an aggravating pollen and we now have air conditioning, central heating, fan heaters, double glazing and insulation so the amount and quality of fresh air in the home has decreased. As soon as there is as light chill in the air we tend to close windows and wrap children up in warm clothes. We also travel greater distances than we would have done even 50 years ago and meet many more people carrying a huge range of infections. This contact with infection is hundreds of times more than it would have been in natural conditions.

- Cigarette smoking is another facet of civilization that has been detrimental to the health of the thoracic lymph nodes. If you look at the lung of a smoker, not only is the lung itself black with soot but the thoracic lymph nodes look like little lumps of coal. One of the adverse effects of smoking is that it partially blocks the lymph nodes so the drainage is poor which makes the resistance to infection poor. A smoker also exhales millions of particles into the air ready to block someone else's lymph system.

- The effect of these modern conditions, sometimes also accentuated by food sensitivities, may well lead to congestion in the nose and throat area. Catarrh, often with bacteria present, may then drain down the trachea into the bronchi and deep into the lungs where it is absorbed by the alveoli and some of the small bronchioles and then travels to the lymph nodes. This onslaught of catarrh may be too much for the lymph nodes to cope with and results in debris filling their spaces and obstructing the passage of fluid through their channels. Such a build up of rubbish also prevents special cells in the nodes, the lymphocytes, from proper contact with any bacteria so they are not able to form adequate antibodies. This weakens our ability to throw off the current infection and lowers the resistance to future infections, so the problem is perpetuated.

The Onset of Asthma

The foundations for bronchitic asthma are very often laid at a young age. At this point, we need to discuss the hereditary factor. There are two aspects to this subject. Although heredity does play some part in a child's vulnerability to asthma, the major cause is usually living in an environment which weakens the lymph system. Given a proper environment there is little difference between the child with an hereditory factor and others. All should be symptom-free. However a child who has asthma in the family does have a greater tendency to acquire asthma if he is brought up in unsuitable conditions. So if a relative has asthma there may be a copycat influence, as the child's subconscious understands that this is the normal way to deal with fluid in the bronchi.

Bronchitic asthma develops in stages and usually has its origins in early childhood. It may progress something like this: a small baby catches a cold and snuffles a little; weeks later he catches his next cold and snuffles more and longer. If the nose and mouth are congested, then the catarrhal fluid may go down the bronchial tube and collect where it causes a rattle in the chest. A further infection causes another rattle, but this time with a wheeze. The next infection brings about the rattle followed by a full blown spasm of the affected bronchi. The asthmatic condition has started.

The Protective Spasm

As we have already seen, small children up to the age of about two do not have sufficient co-ordination between the larynx and diaphragm to cough up mucus and other unwanted substances. As they cannot clear these secretions, the bronchi fall back on the next best thing – they stop them getting there in the first place: the tubes go into a mild protective spasm in an attempt to keep things out and the child may start to wheeze.

So, if a child's lymph system is having to deal with a lot of infection, then each time he catches a cold he will start to wheeze. This wheeze becomes more dominant with each cold until gradually the child's conditioned reflexes get so well established that the slightest sign of any infection makes the tubes go into a spasm anticipating the fluid that is about to come. This is the start of bronchitic asthma. With this particular spasm the tubes close when you breathe out so, although you can take in air fairly easily, getting it out is a problem.

The protective mechanism gets more and more sensitive until eventually any irritation of the nose – dust, pollens, animal scurf and moulds – causes a spasm of tubes. This also affects the membranes of the nose, throat and sinuses. The mild allergies increase the secretion in these areas giving the lung even more fluid to cope with and thus aggravating the condition. It also increases the number of factors that can initiate an attack. Soon only a particle of a previous offender is needed to set off the spasm. Finally, you get a situation where even going out into cold air is enough.

The difficulty is that if, as a small child, your tubes go into a spasm when anything irritates your nose or throat, then this situation persists well beyond the age when you are able to cough up the offending fluid. The mechanism becomes so well established that by the age of five you will still get spasms with any irritation to your nose and throat.

Dormant Problems

In some cases, such as Peter, the symptoms of bronchitic asthma may subside but recur later in life.

Peter, aged 27, had caught a bad cold when he was about nine months old and had snuffled a great deal. He had several colds over the next few months and each time the snuffles got worse. His mother started to notice a rattle in his chest. When he was two and a half, a cold went to his chest, as was now the normal course, but this time he had a spasm of his bronchial tubes – his first attack of bronchitic asthma.

Over the next year or so Peter had further colds, each one going to his chest and each resulting ever more quickly in asthma until the onset of each attack virtually coincided with the start of the cold. By the time he was five, he was beginning to have attacks when he went out into the cold air or met some dust. His constant colds, however, were becoming less frequent and each asthma attack became less severe.

By the time Peter was seven, he just had normal colds and the asthma gradually receded. By the time he was ten it had completely petered out. He remained reasonably fit, although not very robust, until he was 24. Then he had a bad attack of flu followed by bronchitis and a bad attack of asthma. From then on he had been having more frequent and more severe attacks until he came to me for a consultation. Sensitivity tests had shown a large number of substances to which he was mildly allergic. He said that attacks were triggered by cold air, a room full of cigarette smoke or any other irritating substance such as dust in the wind. He was very 'chesty'.

On examination, his nose and throat had swollen membranes and there was some discharge from the sinuses running down the back of his throat. I could hear wheezing over a great deal of the lungs particularly in the lower lobes. There was a number of very large lymph nodes in his neck especially in the area above the collar bone and some spasm of the muscles in the chest area of the spine. There was also considerable water logging of the tissues around the root of the lungs. This was confirmed by X-ray.

Peter had treatment to the lymph nodes in his neck and to the root of the lung and also advice on general health, especially with regards to over clothing, diet and fresh air. After about 15 treatments, he was completely free of the asthma and bronchitis. However, it usually takes some time for the problem to clear permanently and about four months later he caught a bad cold which brought on an attack of asthma. He had another some eight months later but this last attack was very mild and went off very rapidly.

At his checkup a year later, Peter said he'd had no more asthma attacks and was delighted by the fact that he had been the only member of his family not to catch a cold a few weeks before. He also felt much fitter in himself following the treatment.

The reason that Peter's asthma recurred in his twenties was due to his weakened lymph system. By the age of seven a child's lymph system has manufactured antibodies against most of the everyday bugs that he is likely to meet. With so many circulating antibodies, the young Peter was no longer susceptible to infections and it was generally assumed that he had grown out of the asthma.

However, the blockage to the lymph system was still present. While he was fit and resilient he remained free of trouble but as he reached his early twenties and his defence mechanism started to weaken a little, then the sudden attack of flu overloaded his lymph system and brought back the protective spasm causing a return of the bronchitic asthma.

When Asthma Is Not Purely Physical

The psychological aspect of asthma is important to consider. Asthma is a physical disease but it can have a psychological overlay. If a child were about to do something that he really hated and is let off because he happened to have an attack of asthma, then his subconscious will note that the asthma got him out of it. So next time he is faced with a difficult situation he will have another attack. The child does not know that it is simulated – it is the subconscious that is at work, not the conscious brain. This side of asthma needs dealing with at the beginning as it can become more and more crippling – even the slightest thing he doesn't want to do can bring on an attack. Unfortunately so can something which he very much wants to do, because the brain cannot distinguish between something unpleasant and something exciting. The only reason that we can feel excited about someting we want to do is that we have the power of speech which lets us plan future events. Our ancestors, the apes, could not be 'primed'; so the only jolt to their systems was something nasty – such as a fierce lion about to leap. Hence, when we now look forward to something, such as a holiday, this stimulates our adrenaline mechanism and makes our pulse race with the same jolt as the fear of the lion. Unable to distinguish one from the other the asthma sufferer is just as likely to have an attack when he wants to go to a party as when he wants to avoid school.

In an extreme, some children can suffer as many as 10

psychological attacks for every genuine one. So parents need to be reasonably tough and keep their child leading as normal a life as possible in order to minimize psychological attacks. This is well illustrated by the story of nine-year-old Joanna who was such a lively and most attractive young girl that she brightened up everyone's day. She was a delightful child who could twist her parents around her little finger.

Joanna was brought to see me because she was having so many attacks of asthma. I gave her the usual treatment but although the clinical signs got better i.e. the congestion went down, the lymph nodes decreased in size and her breathing sounded better, the attacks of asthma went relentlessly on. This was a great puzzle because there didn't seem to be any good reason why they should continue like this.

The first clue came when I asked Joanna what she was going to do after this session of treatment. Her mother said that they would have to hurry back home as her aunt was coming to stay. Joanna threw a great tantrum and insisted that her mother had promised they would go out to lunch. There was a big argument between mother and daughter. Suddenly the wheezing started and Joanna had a full-blown asthma attack. Her parents looked at each other and said that they would put off the aunt as they must take their daughter out to lunch. Although they had not promised this treat at all, they felt it might help the asthma.

Next time she came to see me, I said that I wanted to talk to the parents by themselves. This is something that I usually never do as I think it is important that children know everything that is going on. But this time I felt that it was appropriate. I explained that, although the attacks were genuine, there was obviously a psychological overlay to the condition: if Joanna knew that they would give in to her every demand under the threat of an asthma attack then they were perpetuating her ill-health.

I stressed that, although it would be very traumatic for

them, it was important to take a tough line. It was, as the saying goes, a case of being cruel to be kind. Her parents phoned up on several occasions saying that Joanna was not well enough to go to school – what should they do? I repeated that they must just harden their hearts and tell the school that the asthma was psychological and it was very important that she didn't get away with it. The parents said that they felt like murderers and I agreed that it was probably one of the hardest things that a parent could ever be called upon to do. 'But', I added, 'If you want a fit child then you must do it'. Once her parents showed Joanna that they really meant it, she got much better. There was the occasional attack but this gradually faded out and in the end she was completely free of the trouble.

It is amazing how quickly the subconscious can stop turning on the attacks if the desired response is denied. It is rather like the story of 'Pavlov's Dog'. If you blow a whistle and put out a bowl of food then the dog associates the sound of the whistle with being fed and so comes to it at once. In the same way, the child associates not going to school with having the asthma attack. If you take away the basic condition i.e. you don't feed the dog when you blow the whistle, then after a few times the dog will gradually realize that he's not going to get any food so he stops coming. In the case of the child, if you clear the basic physical asthma then the psychological overlay fades out because it lacks the reinforcement to keep it going.

Treatment of Bronchitic Asthma

It is my belief that an asthmatic condition is actually made worse by modern medicine. The treatment for asthma has changed quite dramatically over the past 50 years or so. At one time only fairly simple drugs such as aminophylline were available for treating a bad attack of asthmatic spasm. In the absolute extreme people would be given an injection of adrenaline. Such treatments could only be administered occasionally and by a doctor. The aerosols and tablets that can be taken at home on an ad hoc basis were not available.

Nowadays, when a child goes to the doctor with a wheeze he will, sooner or later, be prescribed a steroid and/or bronchodilator sprays to be given as soon as he has an attack. As the disease develops the parents may well be advised to administer these sprays routinely in order to stop the child's sensitivity to particles in the air. If the condition becomes altogether worse, pills of a similar nature may also be prescribed as routine medication. The high level of cortisone and bronchodilator drugs administered to asthmatic sufferers on a relatively long term basis has many detrimental effects:

- These drugs alter the blood supply to the areas affected. At first they cut the blood supply off, then, following that, there is a great increase to make up for the shortages during the active phase of the drug. This brings about the very conditions that the drugs are trying to relieve so they will be needed again to control their own after-effects.
- Steroids lowers the child's resistance to infection as does the increased congestion from the vascular changes so the child is likely to succumb even more easily. With every subsequent infection the body grows more sensitive to the reflexes that close down the tubes, and so the asthma becomes more apparent.
- Treatment with cortisone preparations suppresses the body's natural output of cortisol thus making asthma a potentially life-threatening disease. When I first became a doctor, we always used to say that, however bad the attack of asthma, you could always be assured that at the moment of extreme distress the body would produce a

110

massive output of cortisole and adrenaline to stop the spasm. These drugs can partially suppress the body's natural protective reactions so they may well be a factor in the fatally severe attacks that are now occasionally seen.

Management of Asthma

There are two aspects of the treatment of asthma: care during an attack and management between attacks. If the sufferer has been asthmatic for some time and has been taking steroids or other drugs then the only course of action during an attack is to give the usual treatment. If the attack is severe, then it may be necessary to go to hospital.

However, I believe that the management between attacks needs a complete rethink if the patient is to be able to resume a healthy life without use of drugs. There are several features of my treatment:

- **Change in lifestyle.** It is really important that asthmatic children and adults should be as fit and hardy as possible. If the lymph system is to be restored to full working order we must allow the huge blood supply in the bronchial tree and in the nose and throat to settle down. This means taking the measures described in Chapter 1 and 2 which include: getting plenty of fresh air and exercise, and (children, who are not as prone to cold as adults, cutting right back on clothing) reducing the heating in the bedroom and trying to lead a normal life. This advice is not always easy – but if parents ignore it then the patient cannot be expected to get better, as happened to nine-year-old Ian.

Ian had suffered with asthma since he was three years old. He was originally a healthy baby but by nine months he was beginning to catch a number of colds and getting very snuffly. By the time he was eighteen months, each time he caught a cold he got some bronchitis with it. After a few attacks, Ian became wheezy and the bronchitis rapidly turned into asthma. For a year or two, the asthma only came with colds which then went to his chest. But gradually Ian got asthma if he went into cold or dusty air. Soon he was having asthma even when there was no real reason for it. When I examined Ian there was a large number of tender lymph nodes in his neck right down to his collar bone. He had tremendous spasms and swelling in the muscles of his thoracic spine.

His mother said that she was puzzled how he could be ill all the time when she was looking after him so well. He was never allowed to get cold and was always well clothed. He never went out without some sort of an overcoat. So I explained about the problems of over-clothing and how it was necessary that they try to reduce the level. They seemed to understand and, each time he came to me for treatment, he wore fewer clothes. I congratulated his parents and nanny on how well they had taken my advice on what is quite a difficult thing to do. Sadly, however, with all the treatment and seeming cooperation Ian's condition didn't improve as much as I had expected. There was clearly something going wrong. We looked at the treatment again and spent a long time considering this puzzle. However, two visits later my secretary asked me to look out of the window quickly. Ian had just left through the front door and was being bundled into more and more clothing. He was then driven off in an air-conditioned car. It didn't take much imagination to see why he had not shown the expected improvement.

I had a few words with the nanny and the parents next time I saw them and the message did get through; Ian started to make great strides. After another couple of months he was much better. He did, however, have subsequent attacks, as most patients do, for about three years before he was more-or-less completely free of them. His resistance to infection also became very high.

- **Extra vitamins.** Vitamins A, D and C improve resistance to infections and the ability to throw them off. Vitamin B helps boost general wellbeing. (See page 37 for more details)

- **Check tonsils.** If the tonsils are infected then these need to be removed as the asthma will never be conquered if there is a constant pool of infections and toxins lying in the tonsil. (See page 61) When a decision is being made it is important to remember that the appearance of the tonsils is not as important as the general health of the child and the state of the tonsil lymph nodes.

- **Breathing exercises.** These are very important as, due to catarrhal secretions, an asthmatic person tends to gradually contract the amount of lung that they use. The lung, like all parts of the body, has such a big capacity that we only use a fairly small part most of the time. It is only when we make a major effort that we will actually use most of the lung. It is quite possible to live a fairly quiet life using only a fifth of the capacity of the lung but this fifth should change from one part of the lung to another. An asthma sufferer tends to use only certain parts of the lung and the other parts begin to get less and less usable. Breathing exercises ensure that the whole lung is kept in a fit condition.

- **Physical medicine.** This includes massage to the lymph nodes of the neck, especially the ones above the collar bone, and to the area around the back which is the bra line for ladies. This area is nearly always rather tight in people who suffer from asthma. Such massage can be done at home as outlined on page 26. Ultrasonic waves and surged faradism are used on the enlarged lymph nodes (see pages 26–7 for more details). If the ribs are beginning to become stiff, which happens to a large number of people, then treatment with mobilization to the base of the ribs is very helpful. This assists the range of excursion of the ribs, so improving the breathing capacity of the patient.

On this regime there is usually an improvement in a few weeks. It is then possible to start cutting back on steroids until hopefully they will not be needed. Most children up to the age of around 15 will respond readily and show no further signs of asthma. Treated after that age, patients do somewhat less well and, although they should not have serious attacks, they may still have some wheeziness at times; this would be especially if the patient catches an infection causing bronchitis.

Your Questions Answered

My husband has asthma and I am worried that my 6–month-old daughter will get it. Are there any special precautions that I should take?

Although there is certainly an hereditary factor involved with asthma, as has been discussed above, I feel that too much emphasis is placed on this. After all, there are many people who have a family history of asthma without having it. Asthma is a disease which is acquired, not inherited. In order to prevent this, there are two points which you should note:

- If your child sees her father having an asthma attack, her subconscious may regard this as the correct pattern for any respiratory problems. It is important to minimize everything to do with her father's attacks without making an issue of it.
- In your anxiety to protect your daughter from asthma, you may actually be making matters worse. Although your

natural instincts may be to keep her warm, it is particularly important that you restrict clothes to a minimum and eliminate heating in her bedroom. Prevention of asthma is a matter of letting her grow up in a healthy environment.

I've been told that my son will grow out of asthma by the age of seven, is this true?

If it is bronchitic asthma rather than a true allergy then it is brought about primarily by infection. From the age of around one to seven years old, a child comes into contact with nearly all the common bacteria and viruses that he is likely to meet. So by the time he is seven he will have acquired immunities to virtually all these bugs and will be unlikely to succumb to any further infections. So long as your son is still young and his defence mechanism is fairly strong, then he will appear to have grown out of the asthma. However, if the basic condition of his partially blocked lymph nodes persists then there may come a time, probably in his twenties, when the asthma could return. This is because a bad throat infection or an attack of flu could cause catarrh in the bronchi and reawaken the sleeping reflexes; a spasm would result and so the asthma returns. By this age his defences will be less resilient and his already weakened lymph system will not be able to cope with a virulent infection. If the asthma starts at this age it tends to persist, unless appropriate treatment is given to restore the lymph drainage.

My daughter refuses to wear a pullover or a coat when we are out. Should I insist?

Your child obviously knows what is good for her! Our bodies are designed to live out of doors with no clothes at all. After all, in the extreme, if you put a plaster on the skin for several days it becomes soggy, weak and obviously unhealthy. Clearly, convention says that we must wear some clothes but the less your child wears, the fitter she will be.

We depend on our ability to cool ourselves down by losing heat from our skin. We need its huge area to prevent ourselves from becoming grossly overheated. If your child is too warm then she will have to fall back on the primitive mechanism of cooling by an increased circulation at the back of the throat. This would congest the nose and throat and bring on ideal conditions for asthma. The congestion also reduces a child's resistance to infection so she would become prone to constant colds. This would further increase the likelihood of asthmatic attacks.

Trust your daughter's judgement and leave her coat at home or carry it with you. She'll soon let you know if she is too cold. She's also a lot better without any gloves, ear mitts or hats too. If at all possible and conditions permit, allow her to have bare feet. Shoes and socks are the main cause of many feet problems in later life.

Should I allow my asthmatic son to run around outside when the weather is chilly?

If you protect your child's respiratory tree from all outside annoyances and insults then it will become very weak. If you allow your son to be in air of all types, warm and cold, then he will grow stronger to meet the increased demand. The membranes will strengthen and his resistance to infection will increase so he is less likely to catch colds. An asthmatic child should be encouraged to live as normal a life as possible – and that includes taking plenty of exercise. When you exercise you breathe in more air so any irritants or cold is likely to affect a greater area of lung. If a child is not used to exercise then this can cause trouble. However, if he takes regular exercise then it will have no effect. So it is wise to get him into the habit of using as much of his lungs as possible. Obviously, this should be introduced gradually if your child is not very active.

Should I make my daughter stop playing if she has an attack of asthma?

The answer depends on the severity of the attack. If she just has a mild wheeze, it is best to ignore it and let her carry on with whatever she is doing. However, if she is stressed and clearly uncomfortable, then it is probably better that she sits quietly for a while. If the wheeziness is really bad you may need to use medication: however this should be the last resort. I am not advocating a cruel regime, but it is a big mistake to rush for the spray at the slightest sign of a wheeze. I really do think that if a child can keep going then she should, especially if she wants to. Although the attack may look very distressing to you, she may not be too worried by it.

I've read a lot about the effects of pollution on asthma. How serious is the problem for my asthmatic son?

If your son's asthmatic condition is so advanced that irritants can cause the bronchi to go into a spasm, then pollution can cause a great deal of distress. Pollution is often associated with conditions that filter out much of the ultra-violet light from the sun. This nearly always means that the particles in the air are charged with positive ions which dramatically increases their irritating effect. Pollution can, therefore, play a large part in bringing on a bad attack of asthma. Until the asthma has been cleared with the appropriate treatment, I usually advise the use of a negative ionizer, provided it has the right conditions to operate effectively. And it is best to restrict contact with polluted air where possible. Some people find that masks help, but you should never force one on an unwilling child as wearing one may be quite a frightening experience.

My daughter is about to start nursery school. I'm afraid that she will catch a lot of colds which always bring on an attack of asthma. What should I do?

One of the hazards of children going to school is that they meet a larger number of infections than they are really designed to cope with so they tend to catch a number of colds. If a child has bronchitic asthma then this may well be a problem as colds tend to bring on attacks. When you catch a cold the virus rapidly spreads over the whole of the bronchial tree. If the membranes are a little swollen then secretions will be produced and the natural reaction of the bronchi is to shut down in an attempt to stop them entering the lungs.

Fortunately, with treatment, the tubes will become less sensitive and your child will eventually be able to have colds without an asthma attack. You may well also find that her resistance to infection becomes so much higher that she does not catch the colds in the first place. In any event, once she is in contact with infection at nursery school she will rapidly build up a stock of antibodies to protect her in the future. It is not wise to try and avoid infection.

My child has asthma. Should I try to keep the house free of dust?

This is rather an impossible task. If your child has bronchitic asthma, as opposed to the true allergy, then an acceptable level of dust should not pose a problem. Indeed, too much vacuuming and dusting could stir up the dust and cause more problems than if it was left to lie still. Damp dusting is a good idea as this restricts the movement of the dust. A high quality vacuum cleaner which really filters out all the dust can also be a help. The real problem, however, lies in your child's state of health and measures to improve his reaction to dusts and infections is by far the best course to take.

Does food play a big part in bringing on asthma?

There is no doubt that food sensitivities such as to cow's milk, wheat and certain vegetables can increase a low-grade cattarhal condition. This will worsen the congestion in the membranes of the nose and throat and so make a child more prone to asthma. A good indication of a food sensitivity is when a child either particularly likes a certain food or really loathes it. The only real answer is to elimin-ate the offending foodstuff from the diet. It may then take a year or so after treatment, before the food can be reintroduced without bringing on an attack of asthma. In true allergic asthma the connection is made all too pain-fully obvious by the immediate reaction to even the minutest quantity of the responsible food.

Is asthma a disease of children only?

The basic cause of asthma is the environment in which a very small child lives. If he is subjected to over-clothing and overheating then he will be made vulnerable to asthma. However, it is not uncommon for people in more mature years to get asthma, especially if they have had some respiratory trouble and catarrh before. Sometimes, when a person reaches their fifties an infection, usually flu, suddenly brings on the whole condition with the secretion of extra fluid setting off bronchial spasms. As one gets older the ability to cough up offending substances becomes weaker and so, just as in a small child, nature reintroduces the bronchial spasm to stop the substances from entering the lungs. Fortunately, this soon improves with treatment to unblock lymph nodes, especially in the chest area, to reduce this fluid.

Some older people suffer from a condition known as cardiac asthma which is basically a problem of the failing heart being unable to pump out as much blood as is returned to it. The veins fill up becoming distended, and this leads to water logging of the tissue spaces. In the case of the lungs, the extra fluid may accumulate in the alveoli and irritate the smaller bronchi, these think that the fluid is flowing down into them from the outside and so will go into spasms to keep the fluid out. This is a form of asthma. Once the action of the heart is improved then the bronchial asthma clears.

My son has eczema and I'm worried that he will get asthma. Are the two diseases connected?

Asthma and allergic eczema are both manifestations of a tendency to be oversensitive to allergic responses. If you desensitize an asthmatic child to the substance that is causing the reaction, then unfortunately he may get eczema. It is unusual for this to happen the other way round, but it is possible. My advice would be to look at the cause of the eczema. This may well be damaged tonsils which are putting out toxins that devitalize the skin. Once the tonsils are removed then the skin will clear and the general health of your son will improve. It is also important to maintain a healthy environment; i.e. reducing the clothes he wears to a minimum, allowing plenty of fresh air into the house and turning off the heating in his bedroom. These conditions are not for a child; they weaken his lymph system and this may give rise not only to eczema and asthma, but to other diseases as well.

I've been told that my daughter's asthma is purely psychological. What does this mean?

It is my conviction that asthma is a purely physical disease but it may have a psychological overlay. I have seen children who have as many as ten psychological attacks for every genuine one. Once the physical side of the disease is treated then the psychological overlay gradually fades out through lack of reinforcement.

Other Respiratory Problems

EMPHYSEMA

Asthma causes a blockage of the breathing tubes, especially on breathing out and this raises the pressure of the air in the alveoli when the victim is struggling for breath. Bronchitis also blocks the smaller bronchi causing a similar situation. Both lead to problems with the alveoli in a disease called emphysema. When the bronchi are blocked, air can get into the alveolus fairly easily but it may not be able to get out. This is because when you are breathing in, all the tubes expand slightly allowing in the air which is forced in by the considerable pressure of the atmosphere. When you breathe out and your chest is squashed all the tubes contract slightly so it is harder to get the air out. The net pressure the ribs exert is not nearly as strong as the atmosphere. Now if you cough this puts

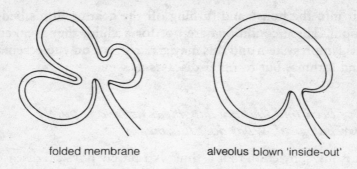

folded membrane   alveolus blown 'inside-out'

Figure 22: Normal alveolus with folded membrane, showing all air close to walls, and alveolus blown 'inside-out', showing air removed from walls.

a tremendous pressure on the air-filled alveolus and you can actually blow it inside out.

Once this has happened, the efficiency of the alveolus in exchanging oxygen is greatly diminished. When the membrane is folded, it takes up a great deal of the space in the alveolus and all the air is therefore close to the membrane for exchange purposes. However, when it is blown out there is a considerable volume of air some distance from the membrane so the exchange of gases is considerably more difficult. As more and more alveoli are blown inside out so the lungs gradually lose more and more capacity to exchange oxygen and carbon dioxide.

There eventually comes a point when a person becomes what is known as a 'respiratory cripple' and such a person can't do much more than sit up and eat. This condition is generally considered to be irreversible. It is widely believed that the effects of emphysema are caused entirely by the blown-out alveoli and that, once this has happened, the tide cannot be turned. However, it is actually the blockage of the little ducts leading to the alveoli which causes much of the problem. Once you can unblock the tubes leading to parts of the lung that are still capable of working then you will often find that a 'respiratory cripple' can lead quite an active life. I have had several patients, like 68-year-old Martin, who have returned to sporting activities once these lymph nodes have been treated and the tubes cleared.

Martin had been a heavy smoker although he had given it up for the last six years. Sadly, he'd had one or two attacks of bronchial pneumonia and this had left him with very limited breathing power so he could no longer ride his horse. He became breathless just getting onto a horse, let alone actually riding one. He found walking very difficult as he lost his breath climbing even the slightest slope. He was told this was emphysema and there was nothing that could be done except a little physiotherapy to get his breathing to as good a state as possible.

I examined him and found that he had a number of large lymph nodes especially at the base of the neck above his collar bone. (These are the ones that drain the upper part of the lung and bronchial tree.) He also had spasms of the muscles in the thoracic spine with the resulting swelling of the tissues in that area. An X-ray showed that he had a number of enlarged lymph nodes in the area around the root of the lung. He was treated with massage and ultrasonic treatment to the lymph nodes in his neck and with surged faradic electricity to the mid-thoracic muscles. He was also given ultrasonic waves to the lymph nodes in that area.

Martin made a very quick improvement as the fluid drained out of the membranes lining the millions of little tiny bronchi that led to the alveoli. This opened up many alveoli that were still actually functional but had not been able to work because the tubes leading to them were blocked. Martin's breathing was so much better that he was able to go riding again.

Four years later he had another attack of bronchitis after an attack of flu and this had left him a bit breathless. With his past history he was very worried about this so he came to see me straightaway. However, after only four treatments he was back on his horse again. That was six years ago and I haven't seen him again but I have had a number of patients from the area who say he is still riding and remains reasonably fit and well.

COT DEATH

A very small baby will sometimes be heard to have a little rattle in its chest as it breathes. It is possibly more common in babies that have been transferred to cows milk shortly after birth. At this early point, fluid will drain into the lymphatics and the rattle will soon clear.

However, if the child is living in conditions that are weakening his lymph system, then he is likely to snuffle more and more frequently and intensely. His bronchial tubes will be faced with an increasing amount of fluid. The tubes themselves may then begin to secrete mucus, as they become irritated by the mucus flowing down, so exacerbating the condition. This rattle on the lungs normally occurs from around one or two months old until around 18 months of age. It has no effect on the child's breathing but it is very easy to hear as fluid moves backwards and forwards around the lung area. I believe that this rattle should be taken very seriously, especially in the first few months. The fluid will contain mucus which can cause severe problems, especially if the child is living in warm conditions with a lot of clothing. The fluid content of the mucus will evaporate as the air the child breathes in and out passes across it, but the mucus will remain. This becomes thicker and thicker until eventually it can suddenly travel down and plug a bronchiole tube. In extreme cases the thick mucus can completely block off a large part of the lung which would lead to a cot death.

This was the case with my own baby son, Mark. When he died, a plug of thick mucus was pulled out like a cast of the bronchial tree. I firmly believe that if parents listened for the rattle and eliminated the mucus then we would see an end to most cot deaths. You can get rid of the mucus at home, or ask your doctor or health visitor to do it for you. Once the mucus is out then the next step is to look at the cause of the problem. I believe that in many cases the baby is sensitive to cow's milk. There are few instances of cot deaths among children who are breast fed for the first few months.

BRONCHIECTASIS

This is a condition that is caused by the smaller bronchioles becoming infected. The infection leads to a breakdown of the wall of the bronchi and as it also affects other nearby bronchi the breakdown coalesces causing an abscess in the lung, which will be in direct communication with the bronchial tree. The main symptom is, therefore, a cough with sputum. As the disease progresses the sputum will become greater in quantity and is often foul smelling. If left untreated more and more bronchioles will become infected and you begin to get an area in the lung where many of the tubes are destroyed. This part of the lung can become so badly damaged that it dies leaving a cavity which continues producing exudate and pus. The person then keeps on coughing this up but unfortunately the pus can spill into other parts of the lung spreading the disease and causing multiple abscesses.

Bronchiectasis can start at a fairly young age, sometimes around 15 to 20 years, and gradually gets worse with time. Special X-rays would then show the affected parts of the lung. Physiotherapy and draining the pus out of the lung by tilting the patient so that the fluid flows out by gravity are useful at keeping the disease under control; thumping the patient's chest to dislodge the discharge (postural percussion) is often employed. Drugs to limit the infection can also be a help. However, where possible, the only treatment is to remove the part of the lung that is infected. If the whole lung is involved then this cannot be done, so there is no permanent relief. However, if bronchiectasis is caught in relatively early stages it can be treated by unblocking the thoracic lymph nodes as described in Chapter 1.

5

A HEAD START

Problems of the Larynx, Skin, Ears, Sinuses, Eyes and Other Parts Drained by the Cervical Nodes

Many people are surprised at the wide range of diseases that can be treated simply by restoring the lymph drainage of the affected area. So many patients say that they have tried all sorts of different treatments for their specific ailment with little joy. Sometimes they have been told that they must simply learn to live with their condition. To me, this is often unacceptable. Provided that the disease has not become too advanced, then there may well be something that can be done to help.

This chapter concentrates on the varying problems that can result from a partial blockage of the upper cervical lymph nodes. When a group of lymph nodes becomes partially obstructed, the whole area is made weaker by the poor drainage but fortunately, it is often only one part of the area drained that develop symptoms. There can be a number of different reasons for this. For example, working in a poorly ventilated, centrally-heated environment, could weaken the sinuses and make them the centre of trouble but probably the commonest cause is a congenital weakness. This frailty of the one area of the body drained by a lymph group could be compared to a design fault in one link of a chain. The chain, representing all the different tissues in one area, would not necessarily break under normal usage, however if put to unusual stress, it would be this weak link that would be the one affected.

As the diagram shows, there are two main groups of cervical nodes. The lower group drains the larynx, the windpipe and part of the lungs. These have a role when a patient has bronchitis or a lung problem and it is interesting to note that in the days before more sophisticated diagnostic equipment, these nodes were taken out and examined under a microscope to diagnose some of the diseases of the lung.

The upper group is the more important however, and it is this large set of nodes which drain the eyes, the nose, the throat, the tonsils, the sinuses and the brain. These nodes are far more often involved in illness than is generally realized. They can become overloaded and partially blocked if:

- A series of lesser throat infections progressively increases the obstruction.
- The tonsils are damaged and continually drain the products of infection into the nodes.
- One sharp throat infection overwhelms the nodes.

As we saw in Chapter 1, this situation results in back pressure of fluid up the lymphatics which causes the associated membranes to fill with fluid and swell. This gives rise to two separate problems which are often present at the same time:

- Mechanical problems due to the swelling of a membrane blocking ducts and filling the spaces they line; and this makes the membrane heap up to form polyps.
- Lowered resistance to infection due to the poor circulation

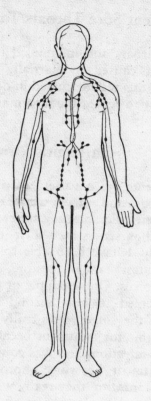

Figure 23

of the tissue fluids and the resulting thick, unhealthy membrane.

These two conditions cause a variety of distressing problems. However, in most cases treatment to improve the drainage can ease the condition considerably by relieving the back pressure and reducing the swelling of the membranes. The main problems associated with poor drainage through the cervical lymph nodes are detailed below.

Recurrent Sore Throats/Tonsillitis

Constant sore throats and inflamed tonsils are a very common ailment caused by partially blocked cervical lymph nodes. As this was discussed in detail in Chapter 3 it is not necessary to repeat the information here.

Laryngitis

Among my patients are a variety of professional voice-users such as actors and singers whose career depends on the quality of their voices. If they suffer from intermittent loss of voice or hoarseness then their job is obviously at stake. Thankfully, I have been able to treat successfully many of our greatest stars and restore, and in some cases improve, their voices. One example of this is a contralto who always seemed to take second place – she was engaged only if the singer they really wanted was not available. She came for treatment because she suffered a number of chest infections and was continually losing her voice. After treatment, her voice improved so much that she became the contralto 'they really wanted'.

Another patient who enjoyed a marked improvement in his career was a tenor who had a beautiful voice but lost it so often that he never dared to come out of the chorus. He had been lucky to get by at auditions and reckoned that, if he was afflicted with voice loss when in the chorus, then he could simply mouth the words. My treatment restored the reliability of his voice and boosted his confidence. Within six months he had been given a solo part in an opera company. He soon rose up the career ladder to become a lead singer and then became a household name when he changed to lighter music.

Our vocal chords have to be shiny and dry in order to

vibrate effectively. If you were to wet a violin string then it wouldn't do so well, nor do our vocal chords if they are abnormally damp. When we use our voice it involves a large muscular effort to make the vocal chords tight enough to vibrate at different pitches. As we have already seen, the greater the muscular effort, the greater the amount of blood needed in the area. It follows that a fairly large quantity of fluid has to drain away from the larynx when it is involved in the considerable effort of singing or acting.

If the cervical lymph nodes are partially blocked then this fluid will not be able to drain away causing back pressure. And the more the effort, the worse the effects of the back pressure. This results in a serious water logging of the vocal chords which impairs their ability to vibrate. The first symptom is squeakiness which turns into mild hoarseness leading on to varying degrees of voice loss.

A single attack of laryngitis is something which is usually dealt with by the local doctor. It is when people keep on losing their voices that problems arise, especially if their career prospects are threatened. The usual treatment is a throat spray either of an antibiotic or an adrenaline-like substance to dry up the throat, often combined with an anti-allergic drug or a combination of all three. In sharper infections the antibiotic would be given in capsule form. However, this is not a satisfactory form of treatment for recurrent attacks, because the sufferer does not form antibodies against the infection. The drying-up drugs cut back the circulation and then tend to result in a huge increase of circulation afterwards to make up for the temporary drought; this in itself can lead to loss of voice and certainly reduces the resistance to a further infection.

In the case of an emergency with a performer, I may recommend using a cortisone spray to the larynx and an antibiotic to help get through a performance. A cold spray on the larynx, for just 30 seconds or so, also helps to decongest it and will offer temporary relief. However, for more permanent relief it is necessary to treat the enlarged lymph nodes above the collar bone and around the larynx itself with massage and ultrasonic waves. Voice training is beneficial. Actors and singers often strain their voices because they are not properly trained and this will put extra strain on the larynx, greatly aggravating the trouble. Proper breathing and projection of the voice is extremely important.

Treatment to unblock the lymph nodes will usually clear the problem permanently and restore a healthy voice. However, on one occasion, the success of the treatment rather back-fired on the patient.

I was consulted by a very famous pop singer who had lost his voice several times when he was on concert tours. The manager said that this was now a serious problem because, when you take a large stadium and you lose your voice, the financial consequences are disastrous. It was becoming virtually impossible to insure him for a concert. I examined the singer and found that he had red, swollen vocal chords and the lymph nodes associated with his larynx were large. He said that he'd had a lot of sore throats in his youth. His tonsils were looking a little unhealthy but the tonsil nodes were not too large. I decided that the problem was caused by the large lymph nodes situated either side of his larynx. He had 14 treatments to these lymph nodes with his voice becoming better all the time. The day finally came when I said that he was nearing the end of his treatment. The clinical signs had improved enormously and his speaking voice was much clearer. His manager agreed and added that the singer had already given a small concert for critics to test his voice out before hiring a larger venue. The unanimous opinion was that the quality of his singing had improved so much that he was in danger of losing his popularity!

Ear Troubles

To understand ear problems it is helpful to look at the anatomy of the ear which is illustrated in Figure 24. The ear is a very ingenious organ and like so many other parts of the body that we have considered, has more than one function. Its primary job is to collect sound, identifying exactly where it has come from, and analysing the sound itself to establish the significance and source.

This is a life-saving feature which enables creatures to isolate the sound of a predator treading on the grass, from all the noises of the birds, the leaves in the wind and the trickle of water. It is this same feature that enables you, in a crowd, to separate what your friend is saying from the noises of the traffic, the hum of conversation and the clatter of cutlery on the plates. Have you ever heard the cacophony of sound that comes from a tape recording of a dinner party?

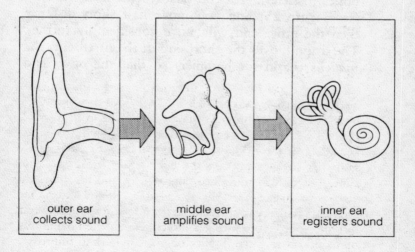

outer ear
collects sound

middle ear
amplifies sound

inner ear
registers sound

Figure 24

- **The outer ear** gathers the sound waves, and, although some of us can wiggle our ears as a party piece, we are no longer able to move them around for optimal collection as can other animals such as a dog. As it travels down the 'trumpet' of the outer ear, the sound is magnified, much as with great-grandfather, who, when hard of hearing, used to present his audience with a trumpet for them to shout down. The sound then vibrates a diaphragm – the tympanic membrane – the ear drum. This membrane separates the outer ear from the middle ear and transmits the sound to it. Although at times prone to infections and eczema the outer ear has problems that are usually easily treated by simple applications, therefore this is outside the scope of this book.

- **The middle ear** has the sole purpose of amplifying sound. This is achieved by a system of 'leverage' of bones (ossicles). If a rod has a pivot near one end (see Figure 25) and you move it a short distance then the other end will move considerably further. The drum moves the short end of the first bone, the *malleus* (Latin for hammer) so that the other end

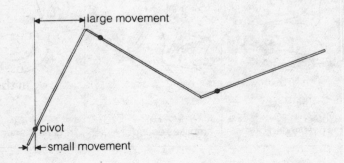

Figure 25

magnifies this movement and, in turn, moves the short end of the second bone, the *incus* (Latin for anvil). The same pivoting arrangement ensures that the far end moves considerably further than that of the original drum. This activates the third bone, the *stapes* (Latin for stirrup), which is planted in the centre of an inner drum, separating the middle from the inner ear, and vibrating it pro-rata.

- **The Eustachian tube** equalizes the pressure between the air outside the middle ear and the air inside. This is very necessary since if the drum is disturbed by unequal pressures, not only will it cause the person to go deaf but it can cause agonizing pain – as any sufferer knows if they go up in an aeroplane. To help illustrate this, picture a simple scientific experiment to determine the atmospheric pressure using a tin can with some thin rubber covering the open end. On a fine day, the air is heavy; on a damp day it is much lighter (water vapour weighs much less than air, so the more of it that is present, the lighter the atmosphere). When the air pressure increases it will push the rubber into the tin. When the air pressure becomes lower, the air in the tin will push it the other way. If you connect a hand on a dial to the middle of the rubber it will tell you the weight or pressure of the air. It is in fact a barometer.

On the inside of the ear drum you have a closed cavity, the middle ear, exactly like the barometer in the experiment, on the exterior is the outside air. Left like this, any change in air pressure would cause problems. If there was a change in air pressure it would distort the drum, wrecking your hearing. Equally, if you climbed up a mountain or went up in an aeroplane so that the air pressure lessened then it would suck your

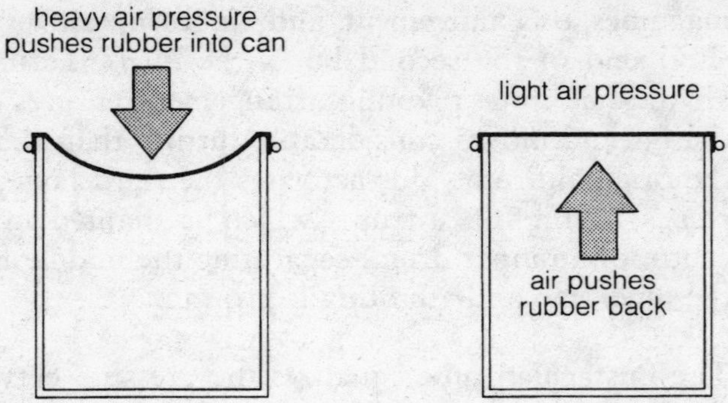

heavy air pressure
pushes rubber into can

light air pressure

air pushes
rubber back

Figure 26

drum out. This is where the Eustachian tube plays its part. It is a small tube which runs from the inside of the middle ear, to the outside air, coming out near the tonsil, and equalizes the pressure between the air outside and that inside the middle ear.

- **The inner ear** consists of three completely separate pieces of equipment, each with totally different functions. Although it is one continuous piece of apparatus the inner ear is another example of how nature has doubled, or in this case trebled up, on functions to make room for so much machinery. It is a complex of interconnecting membranous tubes inside a similarly shaped boney labyrinth (See Figure 24).

1. **Cochlea.** The inner ear is full of fluid which is in contact with the inner drum and is thus vibrated by it. The vibrating fluid transmits the sound to the first piece of apparatus. This is called the cochlea, Latin for snail, because, like a snail's shell, it goes round and round on itself, being wide at one end and progressively narrowing as it goes to the other end. The

cochlea detects the different frequencies in the sound complex and transfers them to nerves that go to the auditory (hearing) centre in the brain.

2. **Semi-circular canals.** The same fluid is used to aid our postural mechanism via the second device in the inner ear which has three canals in each ear (see Figure 27). If you turn one of these canals round on its own axis the fluid will remain stationary; in the same way as if you have a cup of tea with a tea leaf floating on the top, you will find that if you turn the cup round on itself the tea will not turn with it and the tea leaf will stay where it was and not move with the cup.

    Sensitive hairs in a bulge in the canal detect the movement of the fluid, and by combining the information from all six canals in both ears, all in completely different planes, the brain receives very accurate information concerning movements of the head and body. If you look up, the front-to-back canal turns with the head taking the hairs with it, but the fluid remains stationary brushing the hairs. Nerves

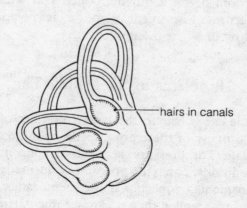

hairs in canals

Figure 27

Figure 28

from the hairs tell the brain in exactly which direction you have moved your head.

3. **Vestibule.** The third piece of equipment is a box (the vestibule) which contains a number of little stones which fall to the bottom when you are standing upright. As soon as you tilt your head these stones move around and sensors in the tiny hairs throughout the walls of the vestibule detect your position and tell the brain. This means that even if you were in a darkened room or on a moving couch you would have a very accurate assessment of your exact position – however slow or slight the movement.

Problems of the Middle Ear

The middle ear is heir to the largest number of problems by far and many of these are directly or indirectly due to an imbalance of pressure between the air outside and inside the middle ear. This pressure is normally equalized by the Eustachian tube but if the membranes lining this small tube are swollen then it can become partially, or less often completely, blocked. Treatment to the lymph nodes in the throat will often largely clear the problem. Quite often, damaged tonsils are continually inflaming the area and making the membranes swell. If this is so then the tonsils should be removed.

Imbalance of Air

If the Eustachian tube is obstructed then this has two main effects:

- It prevents the air from passing freely through the tube to equalize pressure in the middle ear.
- A vacuum may result. Blood is designed to absorb gases from the lungs and tissues, and the circulation in the walls of the middle ear is sufficient to remove a significant quantity. If these gases are not replaced by air passing through the Eustachian tube, then this would cause a vacuum. Sophie's story below shows how this can cause severe earache at times and agonizing pain when there is a large change in air pressure such as going up or coming down in an aeroplane.

Since the age of five, Sophie, aged 11, tended to suffer from earache every time she caught a cold. The pain became more intense and more prolonged on each occasion. She was also catarrhal most of the time and started to get hayfever in the summer months. She had gone on holiday about two months before I saw her and, when the aeroplane took off, she had agonizing earache which continued for half an hour. There was then a loud 'plop' in her ear and the pain suddenly went.

On landing she had bad earache again and was completely deaf for about three hours. She heard a series of gurgles and the pain gradually went. She was given some antihistamine tablets by a doctor where she was on holiday and although she had some earache on the return journey it was not so severe.

When I saw Sophie, the drums of her ears, particularly in the left ear, were very retracted (pushed in) and her throat membranes were somewhat swollen. She had moderate sized tonsils and there were large hard lymph nodes on both sides of her neck. I decided that the lymph nodes were obstructing the drainage of lymph and the membranes lining the Eustachian tube were swollen. This swelling was partially blocking the tube and so stopping the air in the middle ear from equalizing with the outside air. So when there was a dramatic change of pressure the drum was drawn across or blown out causing the acute earache and deafness. Sophie had nine treatments to the lymph nodes and this made her very much better. She did have to come for some treatment over the next two years but after that the trouble completely cleared.

Infection and Glue Ear

One of the most common problems caused by swollen membranes blocking the Eustachian tube is that the infection travelling from the throat up the tube can result in a catarrhal condition of the middle ear: a perforated drum or glue ear.

In its mildest form this causes a low-grade infection and swelling of the membranes leading to a degree of deafness, mainly of high notes, and is often associated with a feeling of discomfort in the ear. This is a very long-standing condition in many cases and is more commonly found in adults. It is a common cause of defective hearing. As in the nose, a slightly sharper infection produces a discharge which can vary from being like water to very thick mucus. Unlike the nose, however, the fluid in the middle ear has only the thin Eustachian tube to drain through and, if the mucus is thick, it may not be able to pass through such a small tube. If it collects, at some point it will raise the pressure sufficiently to burst the eardrum resulting in a discharging ear. Before this can happen, it is greatly preferable for a surgeon to make a slit in the ear to release the pressure when the bulging drum is seen down an auroscope. A surgeon will choose a part of the drum that is capable of healing completely; whereas if the drum is allowed to burst, this often takes place at a site that may not repair for a very long time. Middle ear infections used to be a very serious and distressing problem before the introduction of antibiotics. Today they are not so serious but they are recurrent in many people.

When I saw Lucy she was nearly eight years old. Her mother told me that when she was four, she had a sore throat and some earache. She then seemed quite healthy until the next winter when she had two more sore throats and again rather bad earache. The next year her left ear began to discharge and she felt very unwell. An Ear, Nose and Throat surgeon took out her tonsils and there was some improvement but she still had a tendency to catch a lot of colds. The ear discharged each time.

Lucy had intermittent trouble and was given several courses of antibiotics but the condition did not clear for long. She was eventually brought to me. She had very hard, large lymph nodes as a result of these old infections. I gave her treatment on 14 occasions over a period of four months. At the end of that time her lymph nodes had gone down and her ear condition had greatly improved but was still not completely right. It took about six months for her ear to settle down completely after the treatment. From then on her general health and resistance to infection has been enormously improved.

When the middle ear itself becomes infected or is being

upset by tonsil or throat infections, then this is a prime indication for antibiotics to abolish the infection as quickly as possible to prevent the middle ear from being further damaged by each successive attack.

A discharging ear is one of nature's solutions to the problem of pressure in the middle ear. Another is for the membranes to absorb the water in the mucus which becomes thicker and thicker. This is known as a glue ear. The traditional treatment is for a doctor to insert a grommet into the outer eardrum to allow the gluey mucus to drain out. The plastic grommet is designed so that once the immediate condition has resolved, it comes out on its own after a determined length of time, otherwise it is removed from the drum. This is a very satisfactory treatment as the hole heals and the ear becomes symptomless. A grommet is almost always needed because the glue is too thick for the natural defences of the body to absorb so it needs to be let out; even so the lymph nodes usually remain blocked and the glue ear may well return. It is for this reason that I also recommend additional treatment to any blocked lymph nodes to ensure permanent relief.

I saw Dick when he was four and a half years old. He had become a bit catarrhal at the age of nine months after he had been weaned. He then caught a few colds and seemed to be rather deaf. His mother took him to an Ear, Nose and Throat surgeon who found that his ears were full of 'glue' and put in grommets designed to come out after some weeks. They fell out on schedule but although his ear was somewhat better, Dick was still catarrhal and rather deaf. He complained of earache from time to time. On examination, his eardrums were still somewhat retracted and there was a certain amount of catarrh in his nose and throat. He had a number of large lymph nodes in both sides of his neck. These were treated over a period of about six months, originally twice a week then weekly and monthly. At the end of this time he was much better but still not quite right. A year later, Dick caught another heavy cold and again had bad earache. I saw him and this time, his tonsils looked rather unhealthy. The tonsil nodes were very large. I referred him to the Ear, Nose and Throat surgeon who took his tonsils out.

Dick had two more treatments to the lymph nodes and has remained trouble free from that time.

Tinnitus

When poor drainage upsets the circulation in a particular area of the body nature compensates by increasing the blood supply to the area. This is an attempt to correct the lack of adequate supplies and the build up of waste products. In the case of the ear, some of the increased blood supply runs through the minute ducts across the ear drum and the speed of movement of the rushing blood can sometimes reach such a pitch that it can actually be heard. This distressing condition is known as tinnitus. Sufferers complain of varying rushing, squeaking and other strange noises – sometimes continuously, sometimes at intervals. The apparent sound can vary considerably because the flow, and the number of vessels open, varies but a significant factor is the tension of the drum itself. One of the miracles of many of our senses is that they cover a greater range of sensitivity than you might think possible. For instance, imagine that you are taking a photograph in a room that is poorly lit but has a window opening onto a sunny countryside. In the photo, either the room or the outside will be properly exposed. If it is the room, then the window will be white with little or no detail; if it is the window that is well exposed, then the room will be black.

The eye, however, is capable of showing both at the same time because the sensitivity of the retina varies according to the amount of light falling on it. Where the light is bright the retina detunes; where it is dark, it becomes altogether more sensitive. Go from bright sunshine to the cinema and it will seem quite black and you will stumble around. After a short time, however, you can see quite well as the eye has greatly increased its sensitivity. The same applies to the ear; it can hear a faint whisper, but can also manage to cope with the crash of a full orchestra.

The ear achieves this by a very simple device. If the environment is deathly quiet, a muscle attached to the edge of the drum tightens, stretching the drum very tight indeed. This makes it able to respond to the minutest vibration. If you are at a noisy party, the muscle slackens off and the drum becomes relaxed; it will now only be able to respond to a fairly large amplitude (loud) wave. There is, of course, every gradation of control in between. This explains why noises in the ear are particularly troublesome in a quiet environment and less noticeable in the crowd.

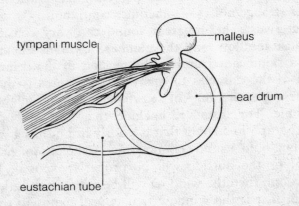

tympani muscle

malleus

ear drum

eustachian tube

Figure 29

The usual treatment for tinnitus is to give a drug called Serc. This improves the blood supply to the whole of the ear and in some cases, by increasing the resistance to infection, reduces the catarrhal condition so it will all settle down. It is a notoriously difficult problem to treat and most people have to resign themselves to living with it. However, I have found that treatment to restore normality to the lymph drainage will often allow the blood supply to settle back to normal thus largely relieving the tinnitus and enormously improving the patient's quality of life. Treatment is very similar to that of the middle ear. However, the muscles at the base of the neck may also need treating because if they are in spasm it leads to a certain amount of congestion upsetting the stellate ganglion. This is a computer that controls the circulation to the ear and can further congest it.

Gordon, aged 63, had had noises in his ears for about three years. He first noticed a high pitched whistle which had only lasted for a short time and he was relieved when it stopped. At first he thought it was some noise from outside and searched around but when other people assured him that they couldn't hear anything strange, he realized that it was coming from his own hearing mechanism.

After a few months he had the whistling sound again; this time it was followed by rushing noises. A few weeks later he found that the rushing noises started up every morning and went on during the day. Sometimes they cleared, sometimes they remained. Gradually the squeaks and rushing noises became more-or-less constant. Gordon said that he noticed that if he was in a crowd with a lot of noise then the sounds were minimal, if the surroundings were very quiet, then they became very loud and obtrusive. They were beginning to interfere with his well-being especially as they were particularly bad at night.

On examination, both of his eardrums were slightly

retracted and red, the left more than the right. He had a number of enlarged lymph nodes in his neck but nothing else much to show. Gordon did have slight trouble at the base of his neck from an old injury. He had treatment to the lymph nodes twice a week at first then at weekly intervals and finally fortnightly. After 16 visits the noises were beginning to subside and he was having several hours when he was free of noises. I saw Gordon again in three months and he was still having noises but they were becoming increasingly less distressing. I gave him two more treatments and asked to see him again in three months. This time the noises were far less. However, he rang shortly afterwards to say that he'd had another cold and the noises had increased considerably. I told him to take antihistamine drugs and the condition settled down fairly well.

After another three months, Gordon said that the noises had largely cleared.

The more recent and intermittent the problem, usually the easier it is to clear up. Although it is not possible to help all cases of tinnitus, around 70% can be greatly improved by treatment.

Arthritis of the Joints of the Ossicles

At the beginning of this chapter we saw that the three bones of the middle ear (ossicles) are connected to each other by little joints to ensure that the transfer of movement be as frictionless as possible. These joints are almost continuously moving as they transmit the sound and so, wear and tear takes place, like in any other bearing. Normally joints repair themselves as they go along, so at the end of each day they are completely repaired. If the repair mechanism is upset by catarrh or poor tissue circulation then arthritis may set in. (See Figure 25)

146

If there is anything whatever wrong with a joint it is called arthritis, in this case the trouble is with excessive wear. The arthritis will start in a very mild form but then the body tries to bolster up the damaged joints by increasing their size with extra bone. If you have a weak hinge on a door you may weld a lump of metal on the hinge to strengthen it but this would unfortunately mean that you would hardly be able to open the door.

The joints are first not able to respond to the considerable movement required for the transmission of bass notes resulting in low note loss of hearing. Unfortunately the joints will also respond stiffly to movement thus obstructing the transmission of the very fast moving high notes so the patient, such as William whose story is told below, may well have high note loss as well.

William, 34, said that he had suffered a lot of colds in his early years and was still a bit catarrhal but that he hadn't had too much trouble for the past 15 years. He had the occasional sore throat and caught a few colds but that was all. However, he had noticed that he wasn't hearing very well. He had his ears tested and was told that he had loss of both the low and high note range.

When I examined William I saw that his eardrums were rather dull. They should be shiny so that when we shine light in the ear to look in it there is a reflection of light back. The membrane lining his nose was a little swollen and there was some discharge. There was a number of enlarged lymph nodes in both sides of his neck. I decided that the joints in the bones of his middle ear had gone a bit stiff which was interfering with the conduction of sound, especially with the bass notes.

William had treatment to the lymph nodes in the neck and gradually his hearing improved. He got about 60% better in two months. I saw him again three months later and he had four more treatments to the lymph nodes which were still somewhat enlarged. During this time his hearing improved very slightly, but when I saw him in a further three months it had become considerably better. After three more treatments the lymph nodes were still not completely normal but we together decided that the amount of treatment that would be needed to obtain a perfect result was not really justified. I saw him finally six months later when his condition seemed stable and his hearing was nearly normal.

Orthodox treatment usually involves trying to clear up the catarrh; first by removing tonsils, if these are infected, and secondly with either pills or sprays to dry up catarrhal conditions. Surgical treatment to the joints of the ossicles can often effect a considerable improvement. My treatment to restore drainage through the lymph nodes which clears the Eustachian tube and improves the tissue circulation and health of the middle ear will usually relieve the problem on a more permanent basis. I use surged faradism to the facial nerve as this greatly improves the drainage away from the ear.

Sinusitis

Chronic sinusitis is a low-grade infection of the membrane lining the cavities. This is a more-or-less permanent state of affairs but every so often there will be a marked flare-up in the condition which is then known as sub-acute sinusitis. This is sometimes brought about by the membrane lining the drain hole of the sinus blocking it so that the infection cannot drain away and thus it increases. Finally, there can be a major infection with symptoms including headaches, pain and usually a high fever. The acute sinus often occurs in a completely healthy person who is momentarily overwhelmed by a virulent organism. It is readily treated by antibiotics and, once it has settled down, may not recur. The first two conditions however, stem from obstruction of the cervical nodes which results in the membranes lining the sinus swelling.

Many patients suffering from sinusitis do not fully understand the role of sinuses so it would be helpful to explain their anatomy and function. Sinuses are actually air passages within the bones of the skull. The skull is necessary for two main reasons: firstly, your brain is such an exceedingly delicate piece of equipment that it needs an egg shaped box, i.e. the skull, to protect it. The second reason is to act as a framework for the attachment of the very large muscles of your head. Muscles are necessary so that you can hold your head up and move it around, but possibly more important, to enable you to move your jaw. The bones of the skull have projections in order to provide an adequate area to fix these powerful muscles. Because of these projections the cavity for the brain is comparatively small in relation to the size of the whole skull. As you can see from the diagram, a considerable amount of the skull is taken up with muscle attachments.

All these bony projections would make the skull weigh so much that it might prevent you from lifting your head up, so they were hollowed out by nature following the best engineering principles. Just as the girders of a racing car are drilled with holes to make them as light as possible, so the bones of the skull are hollowed out. The resulting cavities are the sinuses. A closed cavity would suffer from many problems, as has been discussed with the middle ear, so a drainage tube which can also equalize air pressure is essential.

There are around 60 sinuses in all, most are small like a honeycomb, but a few of the large ones have been given special names. The usual ones to cause problems are the

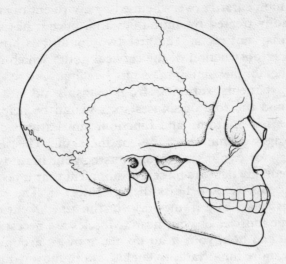

Figure 30

antrum, the frontal sinuses and the mastoid. (See Figure 31)

- The antrum is the biggest of our sinuses. It is the hollowed out bone forming the top of the cheek and supports the big eating muscle (the masseter) that pulls up the jaw.
- The frontal sinuses are the hollowed out bones above the eye. Although we have now lost our ability to move our eyebrows and scalp in the way that apes still can, we retain the large bony attachment of the muscles.
- The mastoid is the air passage through the projection of bone that sticks out just behind and below your ear. This bone fixes the big muscle that comes right down to the clavicle, the collar bone (Latin: *clavicular* = little key), and pulls your head around. It is one of the biggest muscles attached to the skull and needs a very large piece of bone. In the days before antibiotics an infection of the mastoid

150

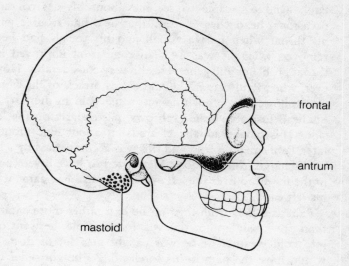

Figure 31

was quite a serious matter because this sinus is so far removed from the outside world and therefore difficult to treat.

Like so many parts of the body, some of the sinuses double up their use. The inner ear and the middle ear are actually built in a sinus, so problems of the middle ear and sinuses are often interrelated. In the same way that the Eustachian tube acts to equalize the air pressure inside and outside the middle ear, the other sinuses have openings to the atmosphere to maintain a constant pressure inside and out.

If the membranes of the sinuses become swollen, these holes can become blocked. The blood circulating in the lining membrane slowly absorbs the air in the sinus or middle ear causing a vacuum. This is one of the causes of the pain of sinusitis.

Paul, aged 67, came to see me about his catarrh and occasional headaches. He said that he'd had trouble with his throat when he was small and his tonsils had been removed when he was 14. This operation improved his throat problems and general health very considerably. However, when Paul was 27 he had a bad attack of flu which was followed by bronchitis and some pain in the part of his head just above the eyebrows, particularly on the left side. This pain gradually cleared but about nine months later, Paul caught a cold and this was accompanied by a lot of discharge from his nose. He started to have severe pain in the forehead over the left eye and he also had earache in his left ear.

Paul said that from then on he had rather more catarrh than previously and at times if, for example, he went out into cold weather or he was caught in a lot of dust, he would have the pain in his forehead. As he got older the catarrh steadily worsened. He had the septum (the division down the centre) of his nose looked at and it was decided that this was very bent to one side. It was therefore straightened by removing some of its cartilage. This improved his catarrhal condition considerably but the headache over his eye remained.

When I saw him, Paul had had two or three attacks of pain fairly close together. On one of these occasions the pain was accompanied by bad earache. He had been put onto antibiotics by his doctor which had helped clear the problem temporarily but it came back after a very short time. He was given antibiotics again; this time they made very little difference.

On examination, Paul had a thick membrane lining his nose and there was some discharge coming down the back of his throat from the nose and sinus area. The area over his left eyebrow was very tender. There was a large number of swollen hard lymph nodes in both sides of his neck, especially the left side. The top lymph nodes were tender to touch.

152

I decided that Paul's main problem was that these lymph nodes were blocked. This was causing poor drainage from the membranes of the nose and particularly from that of the top of the nose which also included the drainhole to the frontal sinus. This little hole equalizes the pressure inside and outside the sinus and allows fluid out. The swollen membrane was blocking the hole and at times this caused a vacuum in the sinus which gave rise to a headache. Paul had 14 treatments to unblock the lymph nodes and improve the lymph drainage. After this, he was about 80% better. When I saw him after three months he said his condition had improved considerably but it was still not quite right. It took a further six months before he was completely free of his sinusitis.

Patients suffering from sinusitis today are treated as far as possible with decongesting drugs, and if necessary, with antibiotics. They may have the pus washed out of the sinus which is then filled with an antibiotic fluid. It is only in extreme cases that the patient is advised to have surgery; this is to enlarge the outlet and then strip out the membrane so it cannot swell and block the hole. Unfortunately this means that you are also taking away a wall that keeps the bacteria out so the sinus becomes more liable to infection. There is a saying that once you have had your first sinus operation then you are going to be a patient for the rest of your life – and it holds some truth.

To my mind, it makes far more sense to attempt to improve the natural lymph drainage. This will allow the membranes to shrink so that air can pass in freely through the ducts and the problem is less likely to recur. Indeed, once the drainage is restored the person actually acquires a very high resistance to infection. Many of my patients have said that they were sometimes the only member of the family to go through the winter without catching a cold. The lymph nodes in the whole of the neck require treating and electrical treatment to the facial nerve (see pages 204–5) is especially helpful. It is also useful to check for any dental problems. If a tooth is projecting into the sinus or has an infected root adjacent to the antrum, this can cause trouble in the antrum and it would have to be appropriately dealt with.

Hay Fever

For many people the summer months are marred by hay fever. The greatest sympathy must go to those people with this condition who have to sit exams as the authorities have chosen about the worst possible moment in the year for these unfortunates. It is called hay fever, because the symptoms are almost identical to a classical fever or cold, with its streaming, blocked nose, swollen and irritating eyes and a general feeling of having a temperature and being unwell. The mind, unfortunately, also becomes affected with poor recall, a lessening of the short term memory and concentration and often, a degree of irritability. The only difference between this and a cold is that with the cold the causal virus is eliminated in a few days and the person regains normal health. With hay fever the poor victim suffers as long as the affecting substances remain present in the air.

Hay fever is almost always a sensitivity or allergy superimposed on membranes which are swollen and excessively irritable because the lymph nodes draining them are partially obstructed. When pollens land and adhere to sticky membranes they further inflame them causing an increase in the local circulation. Unfortunately, the body is intent on warding off invaders at all costs and develops an advance reaction so that one just one speck of pollen will trigger off a total invasion reaction in every membrane within inches of the affected spot. Thus just one speck breathed into the nose sends the nose, sinuses, throat and eyes into an advanced state of inflammation to throw out the invader that never comes. Sadly, the distress to the sufferer is greater from the protection than it would have been from the invader. This reaction is known as an allergic response. It is quite specific to each particular invader.

Around 30 years ago I could say with some confidence that I could relieve almost every case of hay fever by getting rid of a low grade infection in the nose, sinuses and throat. These days, however, there is such a large amount of irritation in the air from pollens of flowering trees, bushes and shrubs whose numbers have increased hugely, both in private and municipal gardens, not to mention the fields of rape, that now treatment to the infection is seldom sufficient.

Conventional treatment for hay fever is with anti-allergic pills, decongesting sprays, cortisone sprays and in extreme cases, long acting cortisone injections. These injections tend to be extremely effective in people with a short season as the benefits last at least three weeks and they have virtually no side-effects. However, my treatment offers complete relief for some and a considerable reduction in medication for others.

The treatment is the same as for sinus trouble. The lymph nodes in the neck need massage and treating with ultrasonic waves; massage also needs to be over the area of the sinuses, cheekbone and down the lymphatics to the lymph nodes in the neck. Surged faradism to the appropriate areas is also usually necessary.

Polyps in the Sinuses

When a person has sinusitus the membranes of the antrum may become very swollen and polyps may eventually start to grow. These polyps can become so large that they fill the antrum completely and bulge into the nose. They can usually be removed fairly simply using a snare. However, unless the conditions which caused the polyps to are improved then they are likely to come again. Treatment to restore the drainage into the lymph system will ensure that the membrane shrinks thus preventing a recurrence. One of the common problems associated with polyps in the antrum is snoring.

> Jo, aged 38, had tried all sorts of remedies to stop his snoring, without any luck. His wife eventually persuaded him to come to my surgery to see if there was anything that I could do. When I examined him, I saw a polyp on the entrance to his left antrum and so I referred him to a surgeon who snared out a number of polyps on both the left and right antra. Jo had several treatments to the enlarged lymph nodes in his neck and was soon sleeping far more peacefully. When I saw him five years later, the polyps had not returned.

Inner Ear Problems

As we saw at the start of the chapter, the inner ear is made up of three separate devices all forming cavities serviced by the inner ear fluid. If the drainage from the lymph nodes in the neck, especially the ones at the top under the ear, is poor this makes it difficult for fluid to drain from the inner ear. The fluid may also thicken a little giving rise to inflammation and irritation of these very delicate pieces of apparatus. The lymph nodes in the neck can be helped at home with massage to the area but they may also need treating with surged faradism to the muscles of the face.

The common problems associated with the inner ear are examined over the next few pages.

Dizziness and Deafness

If the drainage from the inner ear is impaired then this may lead to a low grade catarrhal condition in the semi-circular canals. One effect of this is that the membrane secretes a thicker fluid which does not stay stationary as the head is moved. The brain therefore receives faulty messages from the balance mechanism which tells it that the head is moving although it is stationary. This puts it in a dilemma – if the head is turning, then the room should be seeming to go the other way. As all your other sensors are telling the brain that the head is definitely not moving, it decides that it is the room that must be turning – much as when a train next to the one you are sitting in moves out of the station and you think that you must have started off in the opposite direction. It is the complex resolution of these two conflicting pieces of information that results in the characteristic dizziness – half the person, half the room rotates.

Alice, aged 38, had had her first attack of dizziness two years previously. She did catch an abnormally large number of colds and she had earache with most of these, particularly in her left ear. On three occasions, there was some discharge from her ear but this had rapidly cleared with the use of antibiotics. The most distressing symptom had started after about six months when she suddenly found the room spinning around when she was about to get up.

Alice had five further attacks of dizzy spells, the last two within a few weeks of each other. Her ears had been investigated and it was found that the balancing mechanism of the ears, the semi-circular canals were a bit catarrhal. This made her brain react, as is described above, to think that the room was spinning around.

On examination, Alice had a number of enlarged hard lymph nodes in her neck and these were treated on 17 occasions. At the end of this time the large lymph nodes had virtually disappeared and she had stopped having dizzy spells. She did have two more attacks which were not severe and only lasted for a short while; one was when she had a bad cold about five months later, and the other about two months after this when she had a mild attack of flu.

It was fortunate for Alice that she came for treatment before the condition had become too advanced. As time goes on, the inflammation of the semi-circular canals can lead to the sensitive hairs in the cochlea becoming less effective. This results in varying degrees of loss of hearing.

Caroline, aged 39, came to see me because she had been having so many colds and was very catarrhal. In the last few years, she'd been getting a lot of earache as well. More recently, she was very disturbed because she seemed to be becoming rather deaf. When I examined her, Caroline's nose had a lot of discharge in it and the membranes were a little thick. There was also some discharge coming down the back of the throat.

Her eardrums, which should be shiny, were very dull with a whitey look which meant that they were full of fluid. The drums were also pushed inwards by the pressure of the air on the outside. The bone which joins on the drum was actually moulding it as the drum was pushed over it. Caroline had a large number of hard lymph nodes which could be felt both sides of her neck, particularly on the left side.

I decided that there were probably several reasons that she was deaf: the drum was not transmitting the sound very well; the little ossicles, or bones, were being compressed by the drum so they were not able to transmit the sound very easily from the outer drum to the inner drum; and that there was some catarrh in the membranes of the middle and inner ear.

Caroline had treatment to the lymph nodes in her neck and in the drainage area from the ear and recovered about two thirds of her hearing. The most important thing was that there was no further deterioration in the next year or so.

Another problem that is caused by this catarrhal condition is that the resulting poor tissue circulation in the inner and middle ear leads to an increased blood supply to the area. As has already been discussed, this can lead to noises in the ear or tinnitus. (See page 143)

Menière's Disease

When you are unfortunate enough to have all three conditions at the same time i.e. dizzy spells, increasing deafness and noises in the ear, then the condition is known as Menière's disease. The symptoms are often short lived and intermittent at first, but the noises and the deafness tend gradually to become permanent as the disease progresses.

Peter, aged 57, was walking along the street about 18 months previously when he had a mild dizzy spell. His doctor gave him a thorough examination and took his blood pressure but no reason was found so he put the incident to the back of his mind. However, about a month later the room suddenly began to spin around and he actually fell on the ground. He had two more similar attacks over the next year. Then he noticed some noises in his ears – whistles and hissing sounds.

To his relief they cleared after a while but then the noises returned. When he had his ears tested, it was found that his hearing had diminished somewhat and he was diagnosed as suffering from Menière's disease. Peter was given a drug called Stematil which did greatly ease the dizzy spells but did nothing for the deafness or noises in his ears.

He eventually came to see me and I found that he had some catarrhal membranes lining the outer ear and a large number of enlarged lymph nodes on both sides of his neck. I treated him with ultrasonic and massage and an electrical treatment to re-establish good drainage from the ears. Peter's trouble slowly cleared and after 17 treatments, he was more-or-less free of the noises and had no more dizzy spells.

The orthodox treatment for Menière's disease is largely symptomatic. Drugs to damp down the dizzy spells when they come; and in the extreme an operation to destroy the inner ear when the dizzy spells become unbearable.

Bell's Facial Palsy

This distressing condition occurs when the large nerve, known as the Facial nerve is compressed. This important nerve, running just under the surface, in a little bony canal across the top of the middle ear, controls all the muscles of one side of the face. If the membranes lining the middle ear swell then the lining of the nerve canal may also become swollen thus compressing the nerve and stopping it from working. This is something that often happens

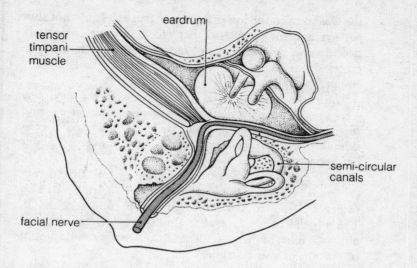

Figure 32

quite suddenly and the sufferer loses the movement of one
entire side of the face.

Usually the condition is temporary and is most commonly brought on by a draught or a bad cold. As soon as
the cold clears up and the associated swelling goes down
the nerve function is restored. However, if the drainage
from the lymph nodes is very poor, then the swelling
will remain to some extent and the patient is left with a
permanent weakness of the facial muscles on one side; this
may be a considerable defect. The main features are: the
drooping of the corner of the mouth, the lower eyelid and,
to a less extent, the facial muscles. It can be most distressing, as the story of Jasmine, aged 33, illustrates:

Jasmine had a very slight cold and when she woke up she
found that her whole face had gone lop-sided. Her mouth
was drooping on the left side, her top eyelid drooped but

161

the weakness in the lower lid meant that she could not shut her eye and the muscles of her face had gone completely flaccid. The sensation in her face was normal but all the muscles that moved her face on the left side had virtually stopped working.

The condition improved a little bit over the next few weeks and she recovered some movement but her eye and the corner of her mouth, which dribbled, worried her considerably. Understandably, she was very concerned about her appearance.

On examination, the eardrum in her left ear looked very catarrhal and was somewhat retracted. The drum was also rather red due to the increased blood supply across it. The muscles of her face were almost completely paralysed although most of them did demonstrate that a small amount of movement was possible.

Jasmine had 17 treatments at the end of which time, the movement in the muscles of her face was about 80% restored. I saw her again in two months for a check-up and the facial palsy could hardly be noticed except when she made certain movements. In another two months the problem had entirely resolved.

The orthodox treatment for patients who do not fully recover is to give support to the structures which have sagged in order to prevent permanent stretching whilst the muscles are unable to function. Muscle tightening operations can also be performed. A more effective result is obtained by treatment to clear the drainage through the lymph nodes. As it is difficult to get to the actual trouble in the canal, electrical surged faradism is almost always needed. This is particularly important as the time element is so crucial; the longer the nerve is compressed the more likely it is to become permanently damaged. After about nine months to a year from the attack, the nerve can start to die from the pressure exerted on it. Although it is still possible to relieve the pressure, you can never restore a dead nerve associated with the brain. So long as treatment is given in time, most people can be relieved of the problem.

Problems Associated with the Eyes

The eye is a special case in the body. The light must be able to pass from the lens through to the back of the eye without obstruction so the eye is filled with a jelly because, as we have seen, a cavity has so many problems attached to it. Unfortunately the jelly is a living material and therefore needs its blood supply and drainage like all other tissues. If, however, it had a network comparable to the rest of the body there would be little space left for the light to pass through, so it has to depend on filtration of the tissue fluid through it, as does the lens mechanism. This works very well provided that conditions are perfect but it does mean that the cells are at the extreme outside limit of distance from the arterial system and their circulation is therefore readily upset. The eye is able to revolve in its socket to avoid the necessity of moving the head all the time to look at something different, this means that there has to be a gap between the eye and the socket. To prevent dust, foreign bodies or bacteria getting behind the eye a loose membrane, known as the conjunctival membrane (Latin: *conjunctivus* = connecting), lines the upper lid. This membrane passes over the front of the eye and then goes across over to the lower lid, which it also lines. It therefore forms a continuous surface sealing off all but the very front of the eye.

Blocked Tear Ducts

Like all mucus membranes, the conjunctival membrane needs constant lubrication to keep it moist and healthy, therefore we have a number of little glands and one large one (the lachrymal which is the tear gland) in the lids of each eye which produce fluid. This fluid has the same concentration of salts as the sea; our cells all originally derived from the sea so they still need that environment for a healthy existence. It also contains an antibacterial substance as an extra aid to warding off infection. We notice it functioning when it pours in large quantities of fluid (tears) to wash away any particles such as a speck of dust or a small insect that may get into your eye.

Lastly, should the eye membrane actually succumb to an infection, the fluid becomes thick and sticky and tends to gum the eye lids together. This is to prevent further infection entering the eye and also to give the eye a rest as, if you cannot see, there is little purpose in moving the eye.

Obviously this constant flow of lubricating fluid has to

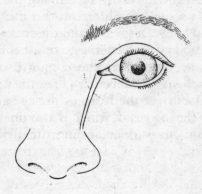

Figure 33

drain somewhere or it would discharge over the eyelid and roll down the cheek, so we have a tear duct which is constantly draining fluid that has washed the eye. The entrance to this duct can be seen as a tiny pimple at the corner of the eye by the nose. The duct runs downwards and inwards and passes into the nose so that the fluid drains backwards into your throat. Only when tears are considerable do they also drain down the nose. Have you not noticed the trumpet of blowing noses throughout the audience as the tears are expelled from the nose after that sad scene in the cinema?

A catarrhal condition of the membrane lining the tear duct can result in a blockage in much the same way as the Eustachian tube in the ear becomes obstructed. The tears are not able to take their usual path and continually spill out, running down the cheek. This can become really troublesome in a wind or cold weather. The orthodox treatment is to try drugs that will shrink the membrane as has previously been discussed. If the condition is too distressing the duct can be surgically enlarged; however this can make the problem worse. The natural reaction of the body to this surgical enlargement is to line the new duct with fibrous tissue which tends to block it off again later on. It may bring about a temporary improvement but the best way of getting semi-permanent relief is to clear the tissue drainage. The treatment is to give massage from the inner corner of the eye down across the cheek bone towards the lobe of the ear and then down towards the angle of the jaw and lymph nodes at the top of the neck; then the general lymph nodes in the neck. This improves the lymph drainage from the lining of the tear duct and can do a great deal to clear the tear duct. Unfortunately again, the lymph drainage can be rather poor and the surged faradism to the outer corner of the eye is often needed to establish a proper drainage.

Blepharitis (Greek: *Blepharon* = eyelid; *-itis* = inflammation)

When the duct gets blocked in older people the fluid dries on the skin and the person begins to suffer sores and ulcers around the eye. This condition weakens the eyelid and it may begin to turn outwards. Such a situation leads to a further increase of secretions in an effort to keep the now exposed inner side of the eyelid moist, so the whole process is accelerated.

> A couple of years previously, Roger, 62, had started to cry rather easily. Anything that upset his eyes such as cold air or draughts made the tears form. This gradually became much worse so that the tears were flowing over the eyelids more or less all the time. As a result he was getting sores where the tears continually drained and his lower eyelid was beginning to turn out a little.
>
> On examination, I found that the membranes of his eyes were very inflammed and the little duct in the corner of the eye had become blocked. Roger also had a small amount of nasal catarrh and there was a large number of hard enlarged lymph nodes in both sides of the neck. I treated the lymph drainage from the corner of his eyes down over the cheek to the lymph nodes. I also treated the lymph nodes themselves and gradually the drainage improved. It was in fits and starts – he would be better for a short time and then the trouble would return. However, gradually, the better periods became longer until he was very much better. Unfortunately he still had tears with cold winds or if he actually catches a cold and becomes catarrhal but the loose eyelids went back to normal.

Thankfully, most people experience a fairly quick relief from the problem once the drainage to the area is improved by treating the lymph nodes in the neck.

Pink Eye and Sties

If the membranes lining the eye, the conjuctival membrane, becomes devitalized due to minor lymph drainage problems then this lowers its resistance to infection and leads either to repeated Pink eye (conjunctivitis) or to infections of the grease glands of the eye lashes, which are known as sties.

Pink eye is an infection of the membrane, most commonly by a particular bacterium called Morax Axenfeld's Baccilus. Other bacteria can be involved. The main symptom is a red itchy eye, commonly feeling as if it has a handful of gravel under the lid. A more severe attack causes crusts of dried mucus on the eyelashes and these can even glue the eyelids together during the night. This may be a single acute disease in an epidemic or a repetitive condition. It is worth pointing out that the typical Pink eye is highly contagious (Latin: *contingere* = to touch) and that many youngsters have a degree of overall congestion that gives the Baccilus the opportunity to get into the tear glands where it can continually re-infect the eye.

The conditions that can lead to the repetitive Pink eye also allow bacteria to invade the ducts of the grease glands supplying the eyelashes. An infection in one of these causes a red swelling, which may be painful, called a sty.

Alexander came to see me when he was 16. He wasn't a very strong person and he'd had a lot of colds in his early years but had grown out of them when he was about seven. He had been reasonably fit until he was about twelve when he had his first attack of Pink eye. He had another attack the following year and this time his eyelids were really stuck together. The condition eventually improved with suitable drops put into the eyes. However, the next year he started getting a sty with mild irritation in his eye. Although this was cleared with some ointment, he then began to get one sty after another.

By the time I saw him he had two sties, one large and one just appearing, on the same lid. He had had them on both eyes but they usually came in the left one. On examination, the membranes of both his eyes were a little red and slightly swollen. There was a large number of firm, enlarged lymph nodes in his neck which went from the top of his neck almost as far as his collar bone.

Alexander had treatment with some ointment to help get rid of the infection and with electrical treatment to help the muscles pump the fluid away from the membrane of the eye down the lymph ducts to the neck. He also had treatment with ultrasonic waves and massage to the lymph nodes in the neck. After nine treatments, the lymph nodes could hardly be felt. His eyes were still a little red and he still had a large sty but this slowly disappeared. He had two more sties over the next two years and a little ointment cleared them fairly rapidly. After that, the problem seemed to fade out and the membrane of his eye no longer looked so angry.

He also commented that he felt a great deal better in himself and that his memory had improved and he was able to think more quickly.

Single acute attacks of both Pink eye and sties can readily be relieved by drops, ointments or in extreme cases, capsules containing an antibiotic. Sties can be helped with hot and cold compresses. The recurrent attacks, which can be very troublesome, are almost always caused by partially blocked lymph nodes and treatment to these will prevent further attacks. This is almost exactly the same as for the blocked tear ducts with massage from the corner of the eye towards the angle of the jaw across the cheek bone and then down over the lymph nodes. It is especially important to take Vitamins A, D and C to build up the general resistance to infection and the ability to throw infections off.

When either of these conditions persist the overall health of the patient needs to be investigated as there may be some underlying problem, such as diabetes.

Detachment of the Retina

If the pressure at the back of the eye becomes too reduced because of the diminished tone of the muscles that wrap around and move the eye, then the eye starts to grow in order to restore tissue tension. All the cells in your body are pressing against each other and so are accustomed to being constantly squeezed. If this pressure is diminished then nature immediately gets to work to restore it. If, for example, you cut yourself; at the edges of the gap there are suddenly a lot of cells which have nothing pressing on them on one side. So these cells immediately start multiplying until they meet the ones also growing in from the other side of the cut.

When the cells meet in the middle, tissue tension is restored so the cell growth stops. In the case of the eye, the lack of pressure on the back of the eye has a similar effect causing the whole eye to enlarge. The retina is rigid and cannot enlarge so this means that it gradually becomes smaller than the eyeball. This results in the retina tearing off from the inside of the eye. Detachment of the retina can happen with very bad short-sight which is also due to the eyeball increasing in size. This is a serious matter which can lead to blindness.

A detached retina cannot be treated at home but must receive the most skilled attention from an ophthalmic surgeon. However, with the agreement of the surgeon, treatment from a competent physiotherapist to improve

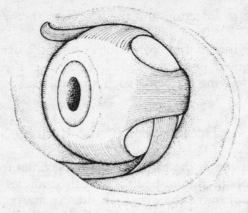

Figure 34: Muscles wrapped round eye and causing pressure on back of eye.

the drainage of the lymph from the area and electrical treatment to improve the tone of the muscles can have a profound and more permanent effect on the end result. I have seen a number of patients who had retinas which were not attaching as well as could be expected and treatment with ultrasonic waves to the eye itself, with surged faradism to the corner of the eye and massage from the eye down the lymph nodes in the neck have caused a fairly rapid improvement.

Arthur, aged 62, had nearly finished treatment to his neck to relieve severe pain around his left chest, when he said that it was a great pity tht physical medicine could not help his eyes. He told me that he had had silicone injected into his left eye because his retina had detached quite badly and this was designed to press the retina against the back of the eye in the hope that it might reattach. The months had slipped by but unfortunately the retina had shown no sign of refixing to the eyeball. I told him that so long as his surgeon agreed that he could have treatment which would both bring the eyeball closer to the retina and greatly improve the repair mechanism in the eye. His surgeon reckoned that he had nothing to lose, so treatment started to the eye with massage over the lymph drainage from the eye, and to the lymph nodes in his neck. He was also given ultrasonic waves for three minutes to the actual eyeball itself. In three weeks the surgeon saw a marked improvement – in a few more months he was able to take out the silicone leaving the retina firmly attached.

So long as the condition is not too advanced and the eye hasn't grown excessively you can restore normal sight or prevent the situation getting worse. Patients with retinal detachments must be managed by an ophthalmic consultant as the mainstay of their treatment, and any other treatment be given only with their permission.

Glaucoma

This distressing condition comes about when there is a change in the pressure in the eye. The space between the pupil of the eye and the lens system is filled with fluid and the rest of the ball of the eye with a completely transparent jelly. This means that the nutrition supply to the cells of the eye has to be achieved without every one being very close to a capillary. To get over this problem the various components of the eye depend to a large extent on filtration: fluid filters through the anterior chamber (lens system) of the eye and then goes out through little ducts all around the edge of the pupil. A very small blockage here is therefore likely to have a very big effect on structures in the eye and produces a disease called Glaucoma.

A change in the angle between the cornea and the back part of the focussing chamber can partly block the exit hole of the drains leading to a build up of pressure in the

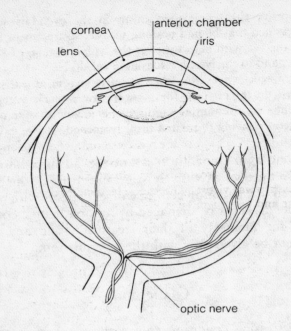

Figure 35

fluid in the anterior chamber of the eye. This is called Glaucoma, and it puts extra strain on the whole of the eye changing the shape of the cornea, further diminishing the filtration angle. The main symptoms of glaucoma are headaches and seeing rings around artificial lights. If the pressure suddenly rises to a dangerous height, the headache becomes severe and the patient feels ill.

Abdul had come over to England for various medical problems. One of these was that he had been seeing rings around lights and after an eye test it was found that he had a fairly mild glaucoma. He was very nervous of having an operation and knew somebody else whom I had treated for glaucoma so he came to see whether anything could be done. I examined him and found that he had a large number of enlarged hard lymph nodes with a history of sore throats when he was a young. These sore throats continued until he was about 19 when he finally had his tonsils out.

Although he had made a good recovery from the operation the lymph nodes draining the tonsils stayed very large as did those draining through the tonsil nodes on either side of the neck. I treated these lymph nodes and gave him electrical treatment to the muscles around his eyes and face, to pump fluid away from the eyes down to the lymph nodes. Abdul had 17 treatments in all, at the end of which the pressure was virtually normal. He came back the following year and needed three more visits. The third year the pressure was normal and he had no further trouble.

If you can improve the drainage so that the fluid in the ducts can drain away satisfactorily and provided you catch the condition at an early stage the pressure will automatically drop to virtually normal. This treatment also uses surged faradism to the corner of the eye and massage from the eye across the cheekbone to the ear and all the lymph glands in the neck. It has been an immense help to a large number of people. It is important to treat the problem in the early stages because if the pressure is allowed to continue for any length of time it will damage the retina permanently, leading to blindness. However, it cannot be stressed too strongly that professional advice from an ophthalmologist must always be sought and followed.

Cataracts

As we have already seen, the eye is a very complicated structure. Unlike the lens in a camera, the eye's lens has varying densities and can change its shape to focus the image on the retina. The lens is made up of living cells

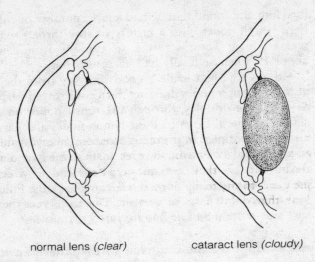

normal lens *(clear)*   cataract lens *(cloudy)*

Figure 36

which depend on fluid filtering through them to keep them healthy. This uses a great deal of energy, so the lens needs needs a good supply of oxygen to remain transparent. If you have back pressure caused by blockage of the lymph nodes, the filtration through the lens can become inadequate and the lens becomes cloudy. This is known as a cataract.

People with cataracts start to notice that detail and colour diminish and the sun and lights become a red dominated glare – rather like Turner's pictures. Turner, in fact, at the end of his life, had advanced cataracts and he painted what he saw. I wonder if he had not had cataracts whether he would have become such a famous artist?

The conventional treatment for cataracts is to wait until the visual defect interferes with the quality of the patient's life and then to remove the entire lens from its capsule. Nowadays it is substituted with an artificial lens. This is a very satisfactory operation. Cataracts, however, can be improved without surgery by treatment to restore an adequate filtration through the lens. The treatment is exactly the same as for other eye conditions with measures to improve the drainage away from the whole eye. In addition ultrasonic waves on the eye itself can greatly accelerate the effect of the treatment.

Alice, who was 69, was greatly troubled by two cataracts which she'd had for around three years. She was a diabetic and at that time they were not very keen to operate on her. She came to me to see if there was anything that could be done that didn't involve surgery. The membranes of her eyes were a little bit swollen and even the membrane over the pupils themselves was swollen especially opposite where the eyelids met. There was a sort of ridge of swelling on the white part of the eye. She had a number of large, hard lymph nodes in both sides of the neck. I decided that, if we could clear the drainage to make it more efficient, this could be enough to improve the nutrition in her eyes. She had treatment with both massage and ultrasonic waves to the lymph nodes in her neck and massage on the ducts from the eyes to the lymph nodes. She then had electrical treatment which made the muscles around the eye pump fluid back to the lymph nodes.

Alice had nine visits in all by which time the eyes were altogether more comfortable and she was not regarded as needing an operation any more. She did however have to come back each year for several years to have three or four treatments to restore the circulation through the eye restored again. She then suddenly stopped coming and I have never actually managed to trace what happened to her.

I can only hope that Alice has had no more trouble. The chance of successful treatment was high, as she came to me at a fairly early stage. It is vital to catch the condition before it gets too advanced as the lens begins to calcify after a time. The situation can be compared to a fast flowing trout stream. If someone puts a dam in the stream the flow of the water slows right up, small particles which would have been carried through, now settle making the bottom muddy instead of stony and clear. In the same way, the cells of the lens begin to go cloudy and later salts start to precipitate out. In the early stages, these can be treated by restoring the lymph drainage, just as the river bed would clear by removal of the dam. However, there can come a point when the mud turns hard with time, and even if you take away the dam the mud would not wash away. So it is with cataracts which then become irreversible.

Epilepsy

This is usually caused by a permanent lesion, or scar, in the brain which, every so often, triggers off a shower of impulses which scatter all over the brain sending it into a state of uncontrolled activty. This manifests itself as an epileptic fit. If all your motor cells are stimulated then all your muscles will contract in a totally uncoordinated manner and, because the activity disrupts all the normal functions, you also become unconscious. The scar alters the brainwaves slightly all the time and this can be seen on an electro-encephalogram (Greek: *enkephalos* = brain; so the word means electrical charting of the brain). At the time of a fit the whole brain function is totally disorganized.

However, there is no explanation as to why the fit takes place at certain times, leaving the brain working normally the rest of the time. Drugs can be given to damp the brain down and these can be very effective in controlling the fits but clearly do have other less desirable effects on the function of the brain. These drugs have to be taken all the time for life.

However, my theory offers a basis for a treatment that can in many cases prevent the fits from starting without resorting to drugs; although sometimes, unfortunately, a greatly reduced dosage is still needed. It is often noticed that a person has attacks of epilepsy if they catch a cold or a sore throat. The reason is that, although the actual defect is present in the brain all the time, the triggering is brought about by congestion in the brain itself.

The lymph drainage of the brain shares that of the throat and so goes through the lymph nodes in the neck. If these lymph nodes are large and have been obstructed through constant throat infections, then they will make the brain more congested whenever they themselves become overloaded; if you catch a cold or aggravate a catarrhal state by cold air, allergy or other precipitating factors then the congestion in your head increases which can set off an attack. I have treated a number of people who have had either almost no attacks, or none at all, after the treatment to the lymph nodes in the neck.

A few years ago I sold my car to a dealer. We were sitting having a cup of tea whilst doing all the various negotiations when he suddenly said that his daughter Roseanne, aged seven, was having bad fits and asked whether I knew if anything could be done. He said he thought it was probably hopeless but whenever he met a doctor he always asked the same question. He told me that Roseanne had been having around 200 fits a year for several years. She had been to Great Ormond Street Hospital and she was on a lot of drugs. He said that when she was heavily drugged the fits reduced but she was not really enjoying life and there seemed to be little hope for the future.

I suggested that he ask his GP to send Roseanne to see

me for a consultation. When she came, I was told that she'd had a lot of colds and sore throats for a great deal of her life. On examination; she had large, unhealthy tonsils which actually had pus in them. She had huge tonsil nodes at the upper part of her neck and a chain of enlarged lymph nodes leading from these down to her collar bone. I explained that these lymph nodes drain the brain; and that it was possible that when the child had a forceps delivery this might have done a little damage to the brain. In itself this might well cause no problems but if the brain became very congested so that impulses shorted from it all over the brain, this would be enough to give the child a fit.

Roseanne had her tonsils out and the surgeon said that they were some of the worst that he had seen. She made a good recovery and then had treatment to the lymph nodes, mostly at home from her mother. She came twice to have some electrical treatment to improve the drainage through the neck area and at the end of that time she was completely changed in her general health. After two or three weeks her doctor said that she could start to let up the drugs and eventually she was able to discontinue them completely. She has had no fits up to the present day.

Temperomandibulitis

The temperomandibular (the temple to jawbone) joint is at the end of a comparatively small bone so it has to be fairly small. However, it also has to cope with the huge muscles of mastication exerting enormous pressures on it. There are a number of factors that can further increase the strain on this joint but it can cope so long as the repair mechanism is in good order.

- One cause of increased strain is when the teeth are irregular in length or do not meet each other correctly. This puts a

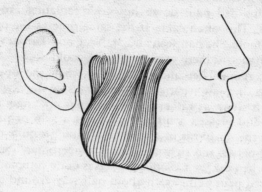

Figure 37

torsional strain on the joint that causes extra wear during eating.

- Another cause is if a person is in a state of anxiety. He then tightens all the muscles of the shoulder girdle ready for a possible fight. The jaw muscles join in the spasm, putting the joint to continuous stress.
- The wear on the joint is greatly increased if sufferers grind their teeth during the night.

The condition can be mistaken for ear trouble, as it causes earache as well as pains up the temple and around the jaw and down the neck (patients sometimes have one or two teeth out, to no avail, because of the pain in the jaw). It is a condition which can cause a great deal of discomfort to patients such as 34-year-old Penny who came to see me because she had a persistent toothache and a pain above her temple on the left side.

Penny said this pain was severe at times and it was especially bad at night. She was obviously in a rather tensed-up state and had a lot of worries. She wasn't feeling very well in herself either. Penny had recently had two teeth out for the

179

bad toothache but unfortunately the pain persisted. At times she also had pain down her neck radiating around her throat. This often came at the same time as the pain over her temple. She had seen an Ear, Nose and Throat specialist who had said there was nothing he could do.

I examined her and found that when she opened her mouth, her jaw went slightly sideways as the jaw joint on the left side was rather stiff. I then put my finger onto the joint and pressed a little; she let out a yelp of pain. This made the diagnosis of temperomandibulitis quite certain.

Big nerves run right across the temperomandibular joint and when the joint is inflammed it is quite common to have referred pain in the teeth about half way around the lower jaw. This is why Penny's pain had not been relieved by having the teeth out. The source of the ache was not the teeth but in the jaw joint itself. The big nerve which runs up over the temple also goes across this joint and, when inflamed, commonly causes pain there.

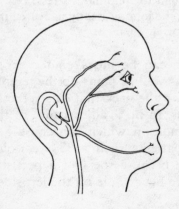

Figure 38

I could also feel that, Penny had a number of enlarged lymph nodes in her neck, especially on the left side, that went down in a group almost as far as her collar bone. She had treatment to these lymph nodes with ultrasonic waves and with electrical treatment to make the muscles on that side of her face contract to force fluid through these nodes. She had the jaw joint gently stretched to get better movement and to help relieve some of the pain. She was also given an anti-inflammatory pill to help ease the inflammation of the joint. After the first few treatments the joint became much less tender. She was given 11 treatments in all and she made a very good recovery. All the pains subsided and she felt much better in herself and generally more clear in her head.

A conventional treatment for temperomandibulitis is to put in a dental plate that evens up the balance of the pressures on the teeth, another is to give tranquilizing pills to lessen the effects of the stress. The best method, in my opinion, is to restore the lymph drainage to the area because that is often all that is needed to cure the condition. Faradism over the actual joint itself is often needed. This problem in the joint is also commonly associated with trouble in the stellate ganglion at the base of the neck, stemming from an old neck injury. This can upset the function of this nerve system resulting in poor monitoring of the joint's repair. If so, this needs to be corrected. My first book, *The Back and Beyond* explains this in detail.

6

ABDOMINAL PROBLEMS

The abdominal lymph nodes are rarely given much consideration. Indeed, you do not often find them on a diagram of the lymph system. When they are discussed it is usually in connection with the part they play in the absorption of fats. Fats are large globules so these obviously need to be kept from entering the smallest blood vessels. They are taken into the lymph system and fed in to the great lymph duct which is known as the cisterna chyli. The abdominal nodes are also noted for their function in dealing with typhoid and paratyphoid bacteria which get into the bloodstream. These latter are not chronic infective conditions and cannot be treated using my form of physical medicine so they are outside the scope of the book.

Generally speaking the abdominal lymph nodes do not get obstructed and cause very little problem. The exceptions are those at the bottom end of the abdomen which drain the bladder and uterus. These can become partially blocked due to:

- **Infections of the bladder.** Infections get into the bloodstream often from our teeth which do not have a totally bacteria-proof connection between them and the gums. Each time you take a bite of food this can cause a shower of bacteria to enter the bloodstream. These bacteria are

182

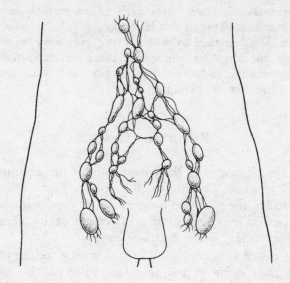

Figure 39

normally dealt with by the filters in the bloodstream, particularly the kidneys. They then pass in the urine to the bladder and thence to the outside world. Unfortunately, every so often a slightly more powerful bacterium can infect the bladder wall causing a stream of debris to go to the lymph nodes lying next to the blood vessels at the bottom end of the abdominal cavity. These lymph nodes can become ever more blocked. This makes the bladder wall swell allowing much less powerful bacteria to invade; so the rate of blockage accelerates.

- **Bowel infections** do not cause as many problems as bladder infections but they can also play a part in helping to block the lymph nodes.
- **Excessive use of laxatives** also has an effect. They increase the amount of the fluid in the large bowel, making conditions more favourable for bacterial growth. This may increase the obstruction of the lymph nodes.

- **External infections**, particularly of the vulva in females, is a common cause of this blockage.
- **An infection such as athlete's foot** may have an effect on the blockage as there is some intercommunication between the abdominal lymph nodes and those that drain the legs (see next chapter).

Recurrent Cystitis

If the lymph nodes in the lower part of the abdomen are slightly blocked, causing swelling of the membrane lining the bladder, then it is no longer able to cope with bacteria and a person may keep getting infections of the membrane. This is cystitis (Greek: *Kystis* = bag).

This distressing condition begins with a feeling of needing to pass urine at frequent intervals. As the infection spreads to the passageway then passing urine becomes more and more painful until eventually many patients say that it is like passing gravel or ground glass. The normal treatment is to take substances that control the acidity of the urine, because most of the bacteria do not like very alkaline water, or in more severe cases, a course of antibiotics. Unfortunately neither of these get to the root of the problem and so the cystitis keeps recurring.

Mary was 37 and came to me because she was having so many headaches. She had been investigated for various conditions – her eyes had been tested, she's had neurological examination and nothing abnormal had been found. When I looked at her she did have a rather stiff neck and she felt tender under the skull bone. This is a very common cause of headaches and indeed was the reason why Mary was having them. After two treatments she said that the headaches were getting better but then she added that the real trouble was her waterworks. She told me that she lived her life doing a dart from one loo to the next, and knew the whereabouts of all the loos on every route she took so she could plan the day. The urgency and frequency of having to spend a penny was spoiling her life. Her doctor agreed to refer her to me for treatment as all his efforts had failed to give her permanent relief. I examined her tummy and found that the bladder area was extremely sensitive to touch. Her abdominal lymph nodes were also large and tender. I suggested that she had originally had one acute infection of the bladder and that this had overloaded the lymph nodes and now the membrane of the bladder was a bit swollen. This meant that every time any bugs were filtered out of the blood by the kidneys – such as from chewing – they settled in the wall of the bladder and so the trouble continued. Because there was so little lymph drainage, she was not producing enough antibodies against all these bacteria and she could not resist or throw off the infection.

She had treatment on 15 occasions to the lymph nodes and to the bladder itself with ultrasonic waves, gradually at longer and longer intervals. At the end of this time, her waterworks had become much less sensitive and she was able to last for longer periods of even an hour without having to go. It was an improvement but it was far from being a marvellous result. The lymph nodes were so much reduced in size that I didn't feel that further treatment would be of any use so I said that I would wait for three months to see her and then reassess the situation of both the cystitis and the headaches. When she came back she said that her waterworks situation had steadily improved and she could now go for at least two to three hours. She was able to face a long journey and a visit to the cinema. After six months, her condition had remained stable.

The main treatment for recurrent cystitis is massage to the lymph nodes in the groin area, particularly on the abdominal side of the inguinal ligament, the big one that runs at the top of the leg from the pubis to the pelvic bone. The other lymph nodes in the groin may need massaging as well because they drain some of the lower parts of the bladder and urethra. You can massage the lymph nodes in the groin area at home but the others are too deep in and will not readily be affected by this. I use ultrasonic waves over the enlarged lymph nodes and surged faradism on the small of the back as this tends to promote a good circulation. Interferential electricity aimed at the base of the bladder can also be very helpful.

In order to regulate the acidity of the urine, potassium citrate is recommended. This can make conditions in the bladder unfavourable for the bacteria and also makes the urine less irritating to the bladder. Patients are advised to drink a lot of water, as much as 2 litres a day, unless they are taking antibiotics. In this case the urine needs to be reasonably concentrated to increase the effect of the antibiotic.

Other advice, such as not wearing unventilated tights and not using personal deodorants or scented soaps can be helpful.

Painful Periods

If the uterus's lymphatic drainage is somewhat obstructed then it becomes a little waterlogged both in its lining membrane and in the muscles of the wall. Under these conditions the blood is not sufficiently liquefied so it may clot and so tends to be pushed out more slowly than usual. The cavity of the uterus is quite small and finds it hard to expel these clots. Indeed, the uterus goes into much the same contractions as those of labour in an effort to get rid of them.

The usual treatment for painful periods is painkillers

and anti-spasmodic drugs to stop the cramps. However, these only offer temporary relief. If other readily diagnosable causes have been eliminated, my treatment may provide a permanent answer by reducing the congestion so the blood does not form the clots and is pushed out by normal contractions. The treatment is virtually the same as for recurrent cystitis. The only difference is that with painful periods there may also be a problem in the lumbar region which needs treating. Symptoms of painful periods may take some time to subside. The body is such a creature of habit that even though the conditions have improved, it is slow to realize that there is no need to produce a cramp to get rid of the fluid.

Selina was 23 when she came to me because she had a painful back. She had a great deal of spasm in the paravertebral muscles in the back and we started treating this. She phoned just before one visit to cancel her appointment because she was having such a painful period that she had to go to bed. When she came back for the next treatment, I suggested that I might look at her tummy as I might be able to help this other problem. On examination, she did have large abdominal lymph nodes and these were treated at the same time as her back. At her three month checkup she said that her periods had been lighter and much less painful. She said that at first the treatment had made the periods heavier but that after a time this had improved.

At her six month checkup she said that although her periods were still painful this could now be relieved by normal painkillers. There is little doubt that the bad back also had a part to play in the problem with her periods. The lower part of the lumbar spine sends out nerves that go to the uterus and control the blood vessels and muscles. If these nerves are interfered with by back trouble this can cause painful periods.

This congestion can also prevent women from becoming pregnant as the fertilized ovum is unable to implant securely onto the wall of the uterus if it is congested. Treatment to reduce the swelling can improve the situation.

Salpingitis

The congestion often spreads as far as the fallopian tubes leading to a condition called salpingitis which prevents the ovum passing into the uterus.

A friend, Elizabeth, who was about 25, suddenly said that she was feeling rotten. She started to shiver and had a real attack of the shakes. We took her temperature and found that it was quite high. She was beginning to get severe pains in her tummy and after having a look at her I was fairly certain that it was a gynaecological problem. It was obvi-

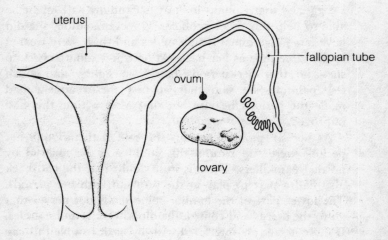

Figure 40

ously an emergency so I asked a friend of mine for his opinion. She had been using an intrauterine coil as a contraceptive and had recently had it removed. When the gynaecologist examined her he found that she had a bad infection and seemed to have a foreign body present. This turned out to be a second coil which had become more-or-less impacted as the uterus had swollen around it. It had then become heavily infected. The coil was removed under anaesthetic. However when she was told about it she said that the coil had been removed the previous week. The true story came out that she had gone to have a coil changed three years before at a clinic and her notes said that the coil must have slipped out at some time because they could not find it; so they inserted another one. The clinic had continued to change the second one – while the other had remained in for the three years. That particular story had a happy ending. She was on antibiotics and made a good recovery.

However, the time came when she wanted to become pregnant and after a time there were no signs so she decided to have a check. The doctor found that her fallopian tubes, which connect the ovaries to the uterus, were totally blocked. She was told that it was the gross infection caused by the coil that must have blocked her tubes and there was no way that she was ever going to have a baby naturally. One day when I was with her, she suddenly burst into floods of tears and told me this rather distressing tale.

I had a look at her and I could feel a lot of firm adhesions in her tummy. An X-ray showed shadows in the back part of the tummy behind the spinal cord which looked like enlarged lymph nodes. She had treatment to these lymph nodes and ultrasonic waves over the area of her ovaries and the uterus. After about 14 treatments, about five months later, she announced that she was expecting a baby. The treatment to the lymph nodes had improved the drainage and had allowed the white cells to remove most of the fibrous tissue and adhesions which had formed to wall off the infection. At the same time because their membrane

189

was no longer congested, the Fallopian tubes were now open enough for an ovum to pass from the abdominal cavity into the uterus. Elizabeth gave birth to a beautiful baby girl.

Food Sensitivities and the Irritable Bowel Syndrome

Food sensitivities have already been discussed on pages 33–34. The lining of the stomach and/or bowel becomes inflamed and forms a kind of low grade allergy to certain foods. The main effect of this is constitutional causing symptoms such as tiredness, hyperactivity and depressions which do not seem to be related to any abdominal problem. In many cases, however, abdominal symptoms are the feature that the patient notices. The main weapon of the bowel against any poison or infection is to remove it by excessive action so the patient suffers from diarrhoea. This creates an additional problem in that undigested food is hurried into the large bowel, where it ferments producing toxins, and these further irritate the bowel. A long lasting condition is thus set up.

Treatment is divided into several sections:

- The main cause of this condition is that the stomach is inflamed. The superior splanchnic ganglion, a computer which lives on the muscles of the thoracic spine, normally switches the acid of the stomach off; when it malfunctions this control is upset and acid pours into the stomach all the time inflaming its lining membrane. This ganglion requires treating as is described in *The Back and Beyond* to reduce the gastritis.
- Food sensitivities need to be discovered if this is possible so that the offending substance may be removed from the diet long enough to allow the sufferer to recover. They can

190

normally be reintroduced cautiously to the diet after the patient had been free of symptoms for about a year.

- The continuous diarrhoea needs to be controlled by drugs that damp down the over activity of the bowel muscles. There are a number of drugs that will effect this result but I have found that Lomatil is much the most effective.
- The lymph nodes draining the bowel, where they are accessible, should be treated with massage but where they are deeper in, with long wave sound. The blockage of these nodes results in a catarrhal condition of the bowel lining which also contributes to the diarrhoea.

Amber came to see me because she felt tired and unwell all the time. About five and a half years previously she had had an attack of indigestion and diarrhoea which had lasted two months. She remembers feeling tired for at least three years before this. From then on she became very sensitive to a number of different foods and had gradually been reduced to eating a very limited diet. Any transgressions and she had diarrhoea for several weeks. At first she had been advised to eat a low fibre diet, but this had aggravated the condition. She was now on a high fibre diet which had helped the bowel condition considerably. Unfortunately the restricted diet was resulting in a serious loss of weight and she was still feeling very unwell.

On examination, she was very thin and had a very pale complexion. Her large bowel and stomach were tender. Her blood pressure was somewhat low. Her back demonstrated considerable spasm, especially in the thoracic spine. Amber then remembered a bad fall over the handle bars of her bicycle eleven years previously when the brakes broke and jammed in the spokes.

Blood tests showed that her red cell count was on the lower edge of what is regarded as normal. She was very low in red cell magnesium and serum chromium. The lymph nodes in the inguinal region were enlarged and X-rays suggested that a number of other abdominal nodes were also enlarged. Finally, the balance of her blood electrolytes was slightly abnormal.

She clearly had HST (hypo sympathetic tone) as described in *The Back and Beyond*, associated with her back problem. This was causing the gastritis and absorption problems. This was treated as described in the book, but with the addition of Zantac to speed up the recovery of the stomach. She was given magnesium, iron and the Vitamin B group to take by mouth and also Lomatil, up to three a day, to control the diarrhoea.

The loose stools stopped almost at once with the Lomatil and Amber began to feel better in about three weeks. However, after the initial improvement further progress was very slow. Three months later she was feeling altogether better and started to look for a job. Her back and indigestion had completely cleared and she was able to widen her diet. This was trial and error and she made some mistakes which gave her diarrhoea for a day or two. Gradually over the next two years she returned to normal except that she still could not eat white flour or tomatoes.

Polyps in the Bladder

A normal membrane should be like marble tiles – flat, smooth and shiny. If the membrane becomes waterlogged it may start to grow little heaps. The body regards these heaps as foreign bodies and tries to get rid of them by pulling them off. They become longer and tend to become a large blob at the end of a thin stalk; this we call a polyp. When a polyp breaks off then its blood supply leaks and the patient passes blood. Polyps may come about as a result of infection but more commonly they just happen. If they are due to infection, treatment to the inguinal lymph nodes will help although the infection needs to be dealt with at the same time (see treatment for cystitis pages

184–6). The polyps that come about for no obvious reason do not respond to this treatment.

7

BACK ON YOUR FEET

One of the general effects of a weakened lymph system is poor healing. Although this can occur with partial blockage to any of the sets of lymph nodes, the point is well illustrated by the story of Frederick whose poor recovery was due to a severe obstruction of the inguinal lymph nodes which are situated at the top of the leg and drain the whole of the leg and a little of the lower abdomen.

Frederick was 19 when he had a nasty accident on his motorbike. His bike was just touched by a car and skidded out of control, finally throwing him off, but falling on top of him. His leg was caught underneath it and he had a very bad fracture. Unfortunately, he wasn't wearing proper protective clothing and his skin and tissues were torn away down to the bone as he slid along the surface of the road. He was in hospital for 18 months during which time the fracture made a very poor attempt at healing. There was still infection present and the tissues never really grew over the bone. It was decided at this point that he should come to terms with having his leg taken off at the knee because there was so little prospect of it healing.

Frederick's attitude was that he would rather have anything than lose his leg and that he would discharge himself from hospital and struggle on as best he could. His father rang me up to ask if there was anything that could be done about this poor healing and I suggested that they brought him along for a consultation. The first thing that struck me was that the tissues all looked very unhealthy, the membranes were waterlogged, the wound was discharging not only some pus but also a great deal of blood stained serum.

Frederick also had huge swollen lymph nodes in the inguinal region. I said that, although I didn't hold out a great deal of hope, if I could improve the drainage from the damaged area by giving him treatment to these lymph nodes and also speed up repair in the area itself with some ultrasonic treatment actually on the injured part of the leg, then I might stimulate some recovery.

After about five weeks treatment with the physiotherapy, the administration of Vitamin B intravenous injections and one gram of Vitamin C by mouth every day, there was a marked change in the whole picture – the tissues were beginning to look much more healthy and were starting to heal and the discharge had stopped. After another two or three weeks the tissues were closing in on the wound.

After four months, skin was growing over the wound and making it look much more healthy. Frederick ended up with a very ugly looking scar but this was better than having his leg taken off. This happened six years ago and he has had no further trouble with his leg since then.

The inguinal nodes can be affected by infections from cuts or bruises to the leg, such as when shaving, by insect bites or minor infections such as athlete's foot, and by ulcers in the leg from more severe injuries. All of these can send a shower of debris up the lymphatics and cause a progressive blockage of the nodes with several consequences.

Persistence of Athlete's Foot

Almost all fungi love dark, damp, warm conditions to prosper; so hot feet inside socks and shoes makes an ideal place for fungal infections to flourish. Shoes and socks act to weaken and dampen the skin of feet particularly between the toes. The spores of the *tinea pedis* (the actual fungi that cause athlete's foot) are probably in the air at times, but may well be present in large quantities on the floor or in a carpet that a sufferer had trodden on with bare feet. The fungi readily spread to the slightly weakened skin between the toes of a new host. The infection is often present for months or even years but if the softened heaped up skin becomes sufficiently weakened it can crack thus letting bacteria infect as well.

Over a period of time enormous quantitites of debris pass up to the inguinal nodes and they can become huge in size. Treating the actual infection can provide relief for a long period if all the organisms are effectively killed, including their spores, and no new infection is encountered. Treatment to the lymph nodes with massage and ultrasonic waves and anti-fungal treatment to the athletes foot makes it possible to stop the infection returning. Massage at home can also be very helpful with this.

Maria loved playing games. She was 17 and she was worried about her very smelly feet. This had been something of a joke at school. She'd been to the doctor when she was 12 and he had diagnosed athlete's foot. He gave her advice about cleanliness and prescribed various local creams and powders but although it got enormously better for a time, it always broke down again. In the end she came to me to find out if I could get a more permanent result.

On examination, she had very large lymph nodes in both

the inguinal regions of the groin and it was my belief that these were obstructing the drainage from the foot and keeping the skin a little bit swollen with low resistance infection. This enabled some spores of the fungus to retain a foothold and when the conditions became ideal these would activate like seeds.

Maria had 11 treatments to her inguinal nodes and they were greatly reduced in size. She had a further course of pills for athlete's foot and some ointment to put between her toes. The trouble cleared up and so far it has not returned.

Recurrent Pain and Swelling of a Single Joint

This is especially prevalent in younger people. If you have a slight strain or twist of the ankle or knee then nature responds with an increased blood supply to initiate repair. However, if the nodes are blocked, this extra fluid has nowhere to drain so the ankle or knee swells. The water logging diminishes the repair mechanism and it takes longer to heal. Even when the fluid has eventually drained away, the ankle or knee is still vulnerable to a jolt, twist or jumping action that would previously have had no effect. Ankles and knees are particularly prone to strains or twists. With each new strain there is a little more damage; and this causes an increase in the blood supply. This makes the situation even worse. Eventually the knee or ankle is weakened to such an extent that it may suffer from swelling and pain for no apparent reason.

Sometimes a person starts the problem in their mid-teens and then by the age of 20 be forced to give up all the activities that make the condition worse. So long as there is no stress the joint now remains trouble-free for some time but at about 40 years of age, it may suddenly become painful or swollen, perhaps on a long walk. The usual treatment is initially rest, then a bandage or stocking and eventually the fluid may be drained with a needle. In some instances it may need surgical treatment. Physiotherapy and exercises are also given, and are probably the most helpful part of the treatment. Except in cases where a mechanical fault is found and corrected, treatments are rarely satisfactory. Most people continue to suffer from permanently weakened ankles or knees.

As the problem is nearly always due to the blocked lymph nodes in the groin, if these are treated then the problems usually clear up extremely rapidly. It is amazing how quickly repair can take place even when there is marked degeneration in the knee.

Phil was a very keen athlete. Unfortunately about 18 years previously he had twisted his knee very slightly kicking the ball when playing football. It became swollen and painful. The swelling had settled down after a week or so and he was able to resume playing. He had no more problems until nine months later when he went on a run, followed by some exercises in the gym, when for no apparent reason his knee became swollen and painful again. Once again it settled with some anti-inflammatory drugs. Only a few weeks later it became swollen again when he was playing football. This became a frequent occurrence and gradually it began to happen fairly early on in the game. He'd even had to abandon the game a few times. Phil's knee had been thoroughly examined and X-rayed at the hospital and it looked very normal. He then had an arthroscopy (looking into the joint with a scope) which was also virtually normal. There appeared to be no good explanation.

This was the situation when Phil came to me. After taking a history about the knee itself, I asked if he had ever athlete's foot, a question that I often ask people with knee troubles. It transpired that he had had it very badly and still suffered at times, even though he had been given treatment. When I examined him, his knee was very slightly swollen but movements were full and the joint was stable. There was no problem that could be found in the knee itself. But when I looked at his groin, I found these lymph nodes were huge as a result of the constant debris coming up from the infection in his toes. This had largely blocked the lymph nodes so that when he sprained his knee slightly on the first occasion, he had had an increase in blood supply to wash away the irritant and speed up repair.

Unfortunately the drainage was by now considerably obstructed. As a result fluid actually overflowed into the knee which upset the mechanics of the knee and also prevented it from making a complete recovery. This was the cause of his problem. He had treatment to the inguinal nodes over a period of several weeks with 11 treatments in all. The lymph nodes never went back completely to normal but they were enormously improved. His knee became much more stable.

Phil has come back occasionally with slight trouble in the four years since I first saw him. His lymph nodes are still too large and they are not actually reducing any more with the treatment so it is possible that he will always have a slight weakness in this knee but he is able to play a great deal of games and sport with only very occasional trouble.

Leg Ulcers

Leg ulcers are caused by a number of factors including poor circulation, varicose veins and diabetes.

Varicose veins cause poor circulation in the tissues of the lower part of the leg. The heart pumps blood out to the tissues all over the body, but expends its energy pushing the blood through the tiny arterioles that finally supply the tissues. For blood to return to the heart, it needs the force supplied by muscles contracting, which squeezes the blood out of the tissues up the veins and so back to the heart. This is described in detail in *The Heart Revolution*. For this pumping to work effectively, the veins must not allow the blood to drain back down them to the very tissues that it has just left; non return valves in the veins ensure the one way flow of the blood. This is particularly important in the case of the legs where gravity exerts a considerable pull downwards on the column of blood trying to travel up the veins.

The breaking up of the veins into short columns means that there is little weight of blood on each valve. If you stand for a long period of time, the blood is not pumped back as efficiently as it would be when you are walking or running; the vein swells a little. This is worse if you have an hereditary weakness in the vein wall. When the swelling reaches a certain critical amount, the flaps of the valves can no longer meet in the centre and the valve ceases to be a barrier to the blood passing back through it. The next column down now receives the weight of both columns which increases its tendency to swell making the next valve fail. There is now the weight of three columns on the third valve so it soon also fails.

As a result the blood in a varicose vein is actually flowing the wrong way down it to mix with the blood brought in by the arteries and then to be pumped up the inner veins of the leg which being supported by the muscles around them always remains healthy; only to flow down the varicose vein once more. This has two bad results: the blood supplying the tissues is half stale so it does not carry nearly the same amount of oxygen and nutrients: and the return of blood from the leg becomes very inefficient as an appreciable quantity of that which is pumped up runs straight back down the varicose vein.

Clearly the tissues begin to look somewhat blue because

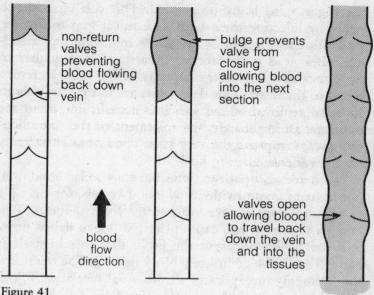

Figure 41

they lack oxygen (blood with oxygen in it is a bright red colour – as it loses its oxygen it gradually turns a bluish-purple colour). The tissues also begin to swell because the fluid cannot get back into the already greatly overloaded veins. Both these factors further reduce the nutrition of the cells. The skin becomes unhealthy and may well break down causing a varicose ulcer. The very fact that it has come about because of the poor conditions means that it has no hope of recovering without help. The immediate treatment for a patient with varicose veins is to wear an elastic stocking or bandage that will collapse the varicose vein and block the reverse circulation – it will also help to squeeze the excessive fluid out of the tissues. The patient should also be advised to keep the legs up above the body as gravity improves the drainage from the tissues. In reality, however, the situation will never improve without

201

the rogue veins being obliterated. This can be achieved either by injecting them with a chemical that makes the walls stick together or by surgically removing the offending tubes. It is important to understand that neither of these measures lessens the capacity of the veins to return blood to the heart – the deep veins are more than able to cope, so removal of the varicosis actually improves the drainage. Unfortunately, the treatment to the veins does not always improve the very poor conditions sufficiently for the varicose ulcer to heal.

There are also patients who have a similar condition, but brought about by diseased blood vessels, for example as seen in some people who suffer from diabetes. Bad injuries to the leg can cause ulcers; so much debris flows into the lymph nodes in the groin that this in itself is enough to almost completely block healing. The treatment that I employ incorporates all the usual measures, but in addition uses physiotherapy to pump fluid actively out of the leg and to unblock the lymph nodes. I also take steps to maximize the health of the patient by ensuring they are not anaemic, give them injections of the Vitamin B complex and also large quantities of Vitamin C by mouth. The physiotherapy is in three parts:

- Long wave ultrasonic treatment given to the ulcer area.
- Surged faradism given to the calf muscles to use the muscle pump to return fluid from the area.
- Massage and long wave ultrasonic therapy to the lymph nodes in the inguinal region (groin).

Desmond, aged 43, came to me with a bad back. In the course of treatment he told me that he was getting very distressed by some ulcers and eczema on the calf area of his right leg. It was both unsightly and irritable. When the eczema broke down into ulcers, of which there were about eight – these were very sore. Despite treatment over a period of six years the problem had slowly deteriorated. I examined his leg and saw a patch of red skin about 14 cm by 8 cm. The skin was very rough and the heaped outer skin had broken down in seven places forming ulcers about 2 cm across. I also found that he had very large lymph nodes in the inguinal region. I suggested that we should treat both the leg and the inguinal nodes.

Desmond had this treatment 21 times and the lymph nodes were greatly reduced down to an almost normal level. The area of eczema had reduced to about one fifth of the area that it had been; the skin was almost normal and there were no ulcers in it. It could not be improved beyond that.

You have now read a description of most of the disorders brought about by a partial obstruction of the lymphatic system. [The list is not absolutely complete but you should be able to decide if this could be the cause of a particular problem.] The next section describes the treatment in much more detail. The information is really intended for physiotherapists as a guide line for them to carry out the treatment.

APPENDIX 1
TECHNICAL TREATMENT

Details of treatment will be divided into sections according to the part of the body – six sections altogether:

Treatment of the head and its associated problems.
Treatment of the throat.
Treatment of the lungs.
Treatment of the abdomen.
Treatment of the legs.
Treatment of the arms.

Treatment of the Head

The first group is sinus trouble, ear problems and hay fever. The treatment is:

- Firstly, massage. This is given down the direction of the lymph system over the frontal sinuses and either side of the antrum to just in front of the ear and then continuing down over all the lymph nodes in the neck. Massage is given in a moderately heavy rotational movement but always pushing the lymph down, first towards the lymph nodes and then from the lymph nodes back to the big vessels at the root of the neck. This should be carried out for about five minutes.
- Secondly, ultrasonic waves. Normal ultrasonic waves are

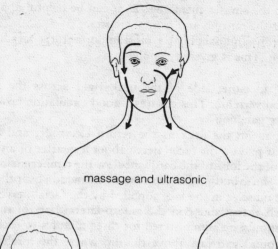

massage and ultrasonic

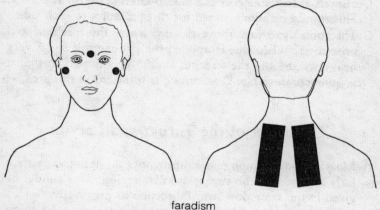

faradism

Figure 42

useful to treat both groups of the lymph nodes in the neck as they tend to break up the debris present. Treatment should be given from the mastoid process down to the nodes just above the clavicle. This should be for about three minutes to each group (which is six minutes in all); longer is permissible but does not do a great deal more good. The new longwave sound penetrates to some extent into the sinuses themselves so it can be helpful applying it over the antrum and frontal sinuses.

- Thirdly, and possibly the most important, the faradic treatment. This is given by applying:

A One pad either side of the neck right across the seventh cervical vertebra. This ensures a good circulation around the stellate ganglion.

B One pad on the neck as the return electrode, and a small circular pad on the facial nerve about a quarter of an inch in front of the lobe of the ear just below the temperomandibular joint. The faradism should cause a contraction over the whole of the muscles in the face supplied by the facial nerve and to a small extent those in the antero-lateral part of the neck. This should be administered for three minutes to each side.

C The round pad just above the dip where the forehead and nose meet. When this is applied the patient will feel a very heavy weight and the strength should be adjusted so that it is quite comfortable. One minute is sufficient in this area.

Treatment of the Throat and Larynx

A Massage to the lymph nodes throughout the neck but particularly the ones in the supraclavicular region. This should be given in the same downward direction as previously.

When the larynx is involved the massage should also be carried over it and back towards the lymph nodes in the posterior triangles. This should be for about five minutes.

B Ultrasonic waves over these lymph nodes and, if the larynx is the problem, over the larynx as well for approximately five minutes.

C The faradism for this problem is given by applying the two long pads over the stellate ganglion for three minutes and then leaving the one pad there for the return. The small round pad is applied to the other two locations; one either side posterior to the angle of the mandible just below the ear, for three minutes either side. This should generate movement of all the antero-lateral muscles of the neck.

Treatment of the Eyes

This is exactly the same as treatment for sinuses except that, following the neck pads, the small round pad is put about 2 cm lateral to the corner of each eye and this should produce a movement of the whole of the extrinsic muscles of the eye which will be seen to 'twitch'. This must be as strong as is completely comfortable and should be for three minutes each side. Then the pad should also be given at the root of the nose. The massage is the same except that it is concentrated a little more on the tissues around the eyes.

Treatment of the Trachea

This usually involves the lower group of lymph nodes in the neck and the ones in the hilar region of the lungs. So the treatment in this case is:

A As above for the throat.
B In addition the long pads should be given either side of the spine over the hilar region for three minutes.
C Ultrasonic waves to the same region for five minutes. If the longwave sound is available this is also very helpful if given over the front of the lung as it penetrates deeply enough to actively help the bronchi and break up mucus. Five minutes should be sufficient for this purpose although in some cases it may be advisable to give a longer period of up to ten minutes.
D Massage over the hilar area also helps to decongest it and possibly reduce any muscle spasm that there may be there.

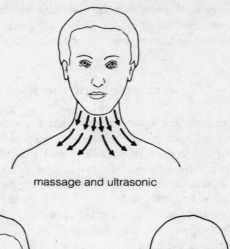

massage and ultrasonic

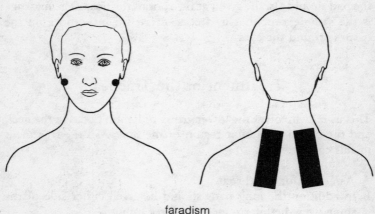

faradism

Figure 43

Treatment of the Lungs – Asthma

This almost always invariably requires treatment to the upper
respiratory tract in addition to the bronchi and lungs. The treatment is the same as above for sinus and throat trouble but is
also given to the lungs. This again involves the long pads either

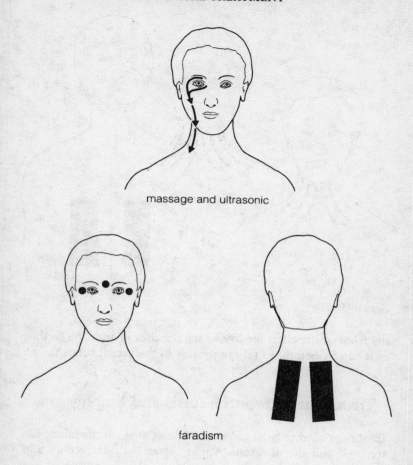

massage and ultrasonic

faradism

Figure 44

side of the hilar region for three minutes, ultrasonic waves over the hilar area for five minutes and massage to the thoracic spine for about five minutes.

With asthma, however, some manipulation of the thoracic vertebrae and ribs in addition is usually necessary. With the longwave ultrasonic it is also useful to give the treatment over

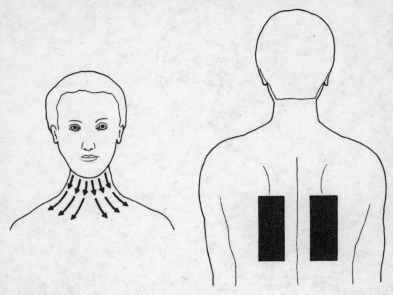

Figure 45

the front of the chest for five to ten minutes in addition to this, as it can be helpful to relieve spasms in the actual bronchi.

Treatment of Bronchiectasis and Emphysema

Treatment need only be given to the lung area; so the hilar pads are used and the ultrasonic applied over the hilar region and over the front of the chest.

Massage and mobilization of the thoracic spine needs to be given.

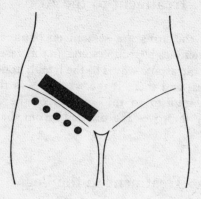

Figure 46

Treatment of the Abdomen

Treatment to the abdomen is mainly for the treatment of cystitis, but could also be given for some uterine problems. It also can be of help to control continual infections of the vulva. The treatment is:

A Massage to the inguinal nodes on the abdominal side of the inguinal ligament. If the nodes on the limb side of the ligament are large, these should be treated also because they do drain the lower part of the abdomen and the perinium. Massage to the mid-lumbar region should also be given.

B Ultrasonic waves applied to the same lymph nodes for about five minutes each side is also helpful. It should also be given to the upper lumbar region of the spine to treat the congestion around the lumbar nodes that lie either side of the abdominal vessels.

C Finally the surged faradism is given through pads in the mid-lumbar region for three minutes.

211

Treatment to the Arms

Problems with the arms are seldom encountered but wound healing can sometimes be troublesome. In this case the treatment is massage and ultrasonic waves to the lymph nodes in the axilla for five minutes, and then, if the wound is in the area of the hand, surged faradism to the muscles of the arm for three minutes greatly improves the drainage from the whole of the arm.

Treatment to the Legs

Problems with the legs are very common. These include infections to the feet, athlete's foot, varicose ulcers, ulcers from poor circulation or wounds which do not heal all of which can cause considerable distress. The treatment for these is:

A Massage given to the lymph nodes on the distal side of the inguinal ligament but it is wise also to treat the ones the other side for a total of about five minutes.

B Ultrasonic waves. The ulcers may well be treated with ultasonic waves for about five minutes, particularly if the longwave instrument is available. The longwave machine can be employed at first the other side of the leg radiating through it and when the lesion begins to heal it can then be put directly on it.

C Faradism to the quadraceps is very helpful at improving the drainage from the leg.

D Quadraceps exercises should be taught to the patient.

E In the case of poorly healing wounds it is also a great help to give large doses of Vitamin C such as 2 gm a day for some weeks.

F Any remedy, such as local treatment or even systemic treatment for the infection whether it is bacterial or fungal can also be employed to speed up the effect of the treatment.

Other than the hip joint, an arthritic knee is the commonest arthritis in the leg, although occasionally a sprained ankle that refuses to repair or the small joints of the foot are the problem. In the case of the knee the treatment is:

A To the lymph nodes in the inguinal region with massage, three minutes and ultrasonic waves, five minutes.
B Surged faradism to the quadraceps for three minutes.
C Ultrasonic waves to the knee itself accompanied by massage and mobilization as indicated.
D Advising the patient to put the leg up as high as possible whenever possible, is also helpful as it improves the drainage.
E An elastic bandage, where applicable, may encourage a better drainage up the veins and lymphatics, and should be employed.

In the case of the ankle, similar treatment is applied to that joint. A common reason for a delayed recovery in a sprained ankle is that the synovial membrane becomes trapped in the joint. In which case, the treatment is to pull the joint sharply apart in a similar direction to the original injury but with the tissues stretched tightly over the joint. This will free the membrane from the joint which gives instant relief. The membrane is often, by this time, oedematous and moulded to the shape of the joint so it can become trapped again necessitating repeating the manoevre. A cold spray and ultrasonic waves, to stop it from swelling, will go a long way to ensure that it does not become trapped again.

GLOSSARY

E.E.G. See Electro-encephalogram.

Abdomen The cavity of the body containing the viscera.

Abdominal Relating to the abdomen.

Acute An illness with intense symptoms and a short duration.

Adenoids Pharyngeal (Nasal) tonsil.

Adrenaline Secretion of adrenal gland that mimics sympathetic activity.

Allergy Heightened reaction to an antigen.

Alveolus Air cells of the lung.

Anaemia - ic Insufficient red cells, or haemoglobin, in the blood.

Antibody Immunising serum protein.

Antigen A substance that stimulates the production of antibodies.

Antispasmodic Able to relieve spasm.

Aorta Large artery leaving the heart.

Appendix A blind, narrow tube leading off the caecum.

Arterial Referring to the arteries.

Artery A vessel carrying blood from the heart.

Arthritis Inflammation of a joint.

Arthroscopy Looking into a joint through a scope.

Asthma Spasms of the bronchial tubes leading to breathing difficulties.

Athlete's foot Fungal infection between the toes.

214

Bacteria Micro-organisms.

Bell's palsy Acute facial paralysis.

Bladder Bag into which urine passes from the kidneys.

Bones of ear Three joining bones which transmit sound across middle ear.

Bronchi Two main air passages.

Bronchiectasis Absesses in smaller air tubes of lung.

Bronchiole Small air tube.

Bronchitis Inflammation of bronchial tree.

Bruise Blood in the tissues from an injury.

Caecum Blind tube off large bowel.

Candida Yeast infection causing thrush.

Capillary Smallest artery that leads to capilleries.

Carbon dioxide Gas produced by metabolism.

Cartilege Glassey, firm, flexible connective tissue.

Cataract Opacity of the lens of the eye.

Catarrh Inflammation of a mucus membrane.

Cellulose The principal constituent of plant cell walls.

Chronic Disease lasting over a long period of time.

Cisterna chyli The dilatation at the beginning of the thoracic duct.

Cochlea The conical spiral of inner ear containing the hearing mechanism.

Conjunctiva - al The mucus membrane lining the eyelids.

Cornea Transparent anterior part of the fibrous coat of the eyeball.

Cystitis Inflammation of the urinary bladder.

Diabetes A disease caused by inadequate supplies of insulin.

Diffuse To extend or spread widely.

Diverticulitis Inflammation of diverticula in the colon.

Diverticulum A pouch off the intestine.

Diverticuloses The presence of diverticula in the colon.

215

Eczema　A non-contagious inflammatory disease of the skin.

Electro-encephalogram　The making of a graphic record of the electrical impulses of the brain.

Emphysema　A condition where the alveoli of the lungs are dilated.

Epilepsy　Fits caused by malfunction of the brain.

Eustachian tube　An equalizing tube going from the throat to the middle ear.

Fallopian tubes　The uterine tubes.

Faradism surged　An interrupted electrical current with a rhythmical change of intensity.

Fungus　Group of plants which lack chlorophyll.

Glaucoma　Increased intra-ocular pressure in the eye.

H.S.T.　Hypo-Sympathetic Tone – an illness that is caused by the lowering activity of the sympathetic nerve system.

Haemoglobin　The pigment in red blood cells that transports oxygen.

Haemolytic　Any agent that has power to destroy erthrocytes – red blood cells.

Hereditary　Transmitted from ancestors or parents to child.

Inguinal　Relating or belonging to the groin, or in the region of the groin.

Inner Ear　A series of membranous sacs and ducts.

Ions　Atoms bearing an electrical charge.

Laryngitis　Inflammation of the larynx.

Larynx　The organ situated at the upper end of the trachea.

Laxative　A remedy to loosen faeces.

Leukaemia　A fatal disease of the white blood cells.

Lomatil　A drug to stop diarrhoea.

Long wave U.S.　As ultra-sonic waves.

Lymph   A pale, yellow, clear (or cloudy) fluid flowing in lymphatic channels.

Lymphatic   Relating to, secreting or conveying lymph.

Lymphocytes   A mature white blood corpuscle.

Massage   Manual manipulation of the bodily tissues.

Mastoid   Air channels in the skull beneath and connected to the ear.

Membrane   A thin layer of tissue which covers or divides a space or organ.

Menière's disease   Dizzy attacks, deafness and noises in the ear.

Metabolism   Chemical processes essential for life.

Middle Ear   Three bones that transmit sound from the outer to the inner ear.

Mucus   The viscous secretion of mucus membrane.

Mucus glands   Glands which secrete fluid rich in mucin.

Muscle pump   The squeezing effect of a contracting muscle to return the blood from the periphery of the body to the heart.

Node   A swelling.

Ophthalmic   Relating to the eye.

Oxygen   A colourless, odourless and tasteless gas.

Pavlov   Ivan Petrovich (b. 1849). A Russian Physiologist.

Peristalsis   A wave of contraction in a muscular tube.

Peritonitis   Inflammation of the peritonial membrane.

Physiotherapy   Treatment by physical means – masssage, manipulation and electrical.

Pink eye   Inflammation of the lining of the eye.

Polyps   A heaping up of a mucus membrane.

Psychological   Associated with the mind.

Red cells   Red blood cells that carry oxygen and carbon dioxide.

Retina   Light sensitive lining of the back of the eye.

Salpingitis   Inflammation of the ovary tubes.

Semicircular canals   Balance mechanism of the inner ear.

Serc   Drug to treat Menière's disease.

Serotonin   A chemical messenger found in the body and brain.

Sinus   Cavities in the skull including the antrum and ear.

Splanchnic ganglion   Sympathetic nerve centre.

Spore   Seed of a fungus.

Steroid   Chemicals related to cholesterol including sex hormones, bile acid, cortisone and vitamin D.

Streptococcus   Round bacterium joined together like beads.

Surged Faradism   See Faradism.

Tinea pedis   Fungus causing athlete's foot.

Tinnitus   Noises in the ear.

Tissue fluid   Fluid bathing tissue cells.

Titre   A measure of the concentration of substances.

Tonsil   Lymph aggragation in the throat.

Toxin   Any biological poison.

Trachea   Windpipe.

Tuberculosis   A bacterial disease mainly of the lung.

Tympanic membrane   Ear drum.

Ulcer   Break in the surface of a membrane.

Ultrasonic waves   A very high frequency sound wave.

Uterus   Womb.

Varicose ulcer   Ulcer in the leg caused by a varicose vein.

Varicose vein   A vein with incompetent valves circulating the blood in the wrong direction.

Vestibule   A cavity in the inner ear with stones in it to enable a sense of posture.

Virus   A microscopic organism.

Vulva   The female external genitalia.

White cells   White cells found in the blood and lymphatic system.

Zantac   A pill for treatment of stomach ulcers.

INDEX

abdomen, treatment of the, 211
abdominal adenitis, 89
abscess
  appendix, 84
  lungs, 125
adenoids, 16, 61, 81–2
adrenaline, 110, 111
air
  stale, 52
  warmed, 52–3
air conditioning, and positive
  ionization, 53
alcohol, 37
allergic asthma, 96–7, 119
allergies
  allergic asthma, 96–7, 119
  hay fever, 154–5
  see also food sensitivities
alveoli, 99–100, 122
aminophylline, 109–10
ankle
  sprained, 213
  swollen, 24
anti-inflammatory drugs, 28–9
antibiotics, 29–33
  adverse effects, 32
  course of treatment, 30–1, 32
  effectiveness, 29, 30
  effects on essential bacteria, 32–3
  over long periods, 32
  over-use, 25, 29
  strength of dosage, 31
antibodies, 25, 55, 57, 63
antibody response, 24, 83
anxiety states, 37
appendicitis see chronic appendicitis
appendix, 13, 16, 17, 18, 61, 82–94
  abscessed, 84
  infected, 83–4
  scarring, 83, 84
  see also chronic appendicitis
appetite loss, 88
arms, treatment to the, 212
arthritis
  arthritic knee, 213
  of the joints of the ossicles, 146–8
asthma, 95–121

in adults, 119–20
allergic asthma, 96–7, 119
and allergic eczema, 120–1
benefits of exercise, 116–17
cardiac asthma, 120
in children, 98, 103–5, 107–9,
  114–19, 120–1
food sensitivities, 119
'growing out of', 115
hereditary factor, 14–15, 103, 114
house cleaning and, 118–19
increase in numbers of asthmatics, 95
management of, 111–14
masks, 118
over-clothing and congestion, 115–16
pollution and, 17–18
psychological aspect, 107–9, 121
questions and concerns, 114–21
treatment, 209–10
see also bronchitic asthma
asthma, management of, 111–14
  breathing exercises, 113
  in children, 114
  dietary factors, 119
  house cleaning and, 118–19
  lifestyle, change in, 111–13
  massage, 113
  physical medicine, 113–14
  tonsils, checking the, 113
  vitamin supplements, 113
athlete's foot, 20, 184, 196–7

babies
  and body temperature, 44, 45, 49–50
  breast feeding, 34, 57–8, 125
  cot deaths, 124–5
  immunity, development of, 57–8
  lymph system in, 41
  sensitivity to cow's milk, 125
back pain, 37, 38, 42
bacteria, 15, 16, 23, 24, 25, 30, 31
  in the appendix, 84
  in the bowel, 94
  and dental problems, 36
  essential, 32–3
  in food, 55, 56, 57, 71
  in the tonsils, 62, 63, 64

219